Basic Surgical Instrumentation

MARY F. SMITH, R.N., B.S.N., CNOR

Program Director
United Medical Center
School of Surgical Technology
Moline, Illinois

JOETTE L. STEHN, R.N., A.D.N., CST

Clinical Instructor
United Medical Center
School of Surgical Technology
Moline, Illinois

W. B. SAUNDERS COMPANY
A Division of Harcourt Brace & Company
Philadelphia   London   Toronto   Montreal   Sydney   Tokyo

W.B. SAUNDERS COMPANY
A Division of
Harcourt Brace & Company

The Curtis Center
Independence Square West
Philadelphia, Pennsylvania 19106

Library of Congress Cataloging-in-Publication Data

Smith, Mary F., R.N.
    Basic surgical instrumentation / Mary F. Smith, Joette
Stehn.
        p.   cm.
    Includes index.

    ISBN 0-7216-4211-X

    1. Surgical instruments and apparatus.   I. Stehn,
Joette.   II. Title
    [DNLM: 1. Surgical Equipment.   2. Surgical
Instruments.   W 26   S655b]
RD71.S584   1993
617′.9178—dc20
DNLM/DLC   92-49933

Basic Surgical Instrumentation   ISBN 0-7216-4211-X

Printed in the United States of America.

Last digit is the print number: 9   8   7   6   5   4   3   2

We would like to dedicate this book to our families.

*With their encouragement and understanding and relinquishing of family time,
we are able to see a dream become a reality.*

Thank you, Danny, Elisabeth, Rebecca, Andrew [JLS].
Thank you, Al, Brad, Jean, Heath, Chris [MFS].

Preface

Basic Surgical Instrumentation is meant to be a basic point of reference for inexperienced personnel in surgical departments and allied supporting areas.

As OR technology evolves into a complex maze of patient care procedures and high technology instrumentation, it is increasingly necessary to have a very basic instrument reference book.

After acquiring knowledge of basic instruments and sets, it is easier to build knowledge in specialty areas.

With the highly mobile surgical department personnel today, it is imperative that the instrument book be as comprehensive as possible, yet remain an easy, quick reference when needed.

Because surgical department and allied supporting personnel must function rapidly and maintain a high degree of competency in recognizing the names and identifying the instruments for handling, this book is intended to speed the recognition and identification process.

Acknowledgments

Special thanks to Barry Halm, CEO, United Medical Center, Moline, Illinois, who encouraged our efforts and enthusiastically supported our endeavors.

To Steve Kosmach, RN, BSN, and the wonderful staff in the Central Processing Department who assisted us with photographs. Without the cooperation of the staff of the CPD, our project would not have been possible.

To the United Medical Center Surgical Technology Class of 1992 who supported us in our down days, tolerated us when we worked long hours, and shared our anxieties for six months.

To the United Medical Center Surgery Staff who served as unofficial technical advisors when we needed a consultation.

We also wish to extend our thanks to the following companies for their excellent resource materials:

Acufex Microsurgical, Inc.
130 Forbes Boulevard
Mansfield, MA 02048

Aesculap, Inc.
1000 Gateway Boulevard
South San Francisco, CA 94080

Baxter Healthcare Corporation
1500 Waukegan Road
McGaw Park, IL 60085
V. Mueller Division

Becton Dickinson
One Becton Drive
Franklin Lakes, NJ 07417

Codman & Shurtleff, Inc.
41 Pacella Park
Randolph, MA 02368

Linvatec (Weck Endoscopy)
PO Box
12600 Weck Drive
Research Triangle Park, NC 27709

Miltex Instrument Company, Inc.
6 Ohio Drive
Lake Success, NY 11042

Pilling-Rusch
420 Delaware Drive
Fort Washington, PA 19034

Richard Wolf Medical Instruments
353 Corporate Woods Parkway
Vernon Hills, IL 60061

Storz
3365 Tree Court Industrial Boulevard
St. Louis, MO 63122

Zimmer Schilling Associates, Inc.
5117 Jersey Ridge Road
Davenport, IA 52807

Contents

CHAPTER

1

Introduction

Our goal in preparing this book is to provide a basis on which an individual can build knowledge of instruments used in surgical procedures. We have attempted to show basic instruments to give the person who is new to the arena of surgical instrumentation the fundamentals without an overload of specialty instruments.

It is difficult to decide how "basic" some specialty areas have become. We have not included the complex area of orthopedic fixation since this can be considered an entire specialty area. Many manufacturers supply fixation components of similar properties, and the instruments used depend on each surgeon's preference. We do, however, provide information on basic orthopedic instrumentation used in hip and knee implant procedures.

Geographic nomenclature, surgeon preferences, regional custom manufacturers, and suppliers result in the use of multiple names for the same instruments, which will continue to be used and pose problems for the novice instrument user. Favorite names for instruments have a way of being integrated into the surgical instrumentation arena quite easily in our mobile and information-sharing society.

It is extremely difficult to design basic major and minor instrument sets without leaving out that one instrument that one could reasonably argue that "all the surgeons use." The basic instruments presented here are intended to serve as a guide to enable individuals to meet the needs of their institutions.

INSTRUMENT MECHANICS

History of Instrument Mechanics

Proof that surgical instrumentation began hundreds of years ago has been determined by the items found by archaeologists throughout the world. One of the earliest identified tools is a simple sharp device used to penetrate the skull. This act of "trephining," creating a hole through the skull, was performed to release the demons causing illness or unacceptable behavior by the patient. These penetrating devices were usually made of sharpened flint rock. The earliest surgical instruments were made of the various substances available to the most skilled craftsman in the area, such as copper, iron, glass, ivory, and wood. Virtually any substance that could be molded or formed to the specifications of the surgeon's needs was hand made into a multipurpose surgical instrument.

However, the number of instruments available to the surgeon was extremely limited. A surgeon of the 1800s packed his bag with ordinary kitchen utensils and his own special pocket knife and saw. As acceptance of the surgeon's skills increased, the demand for specialized instruments increased. A surgeon's own custom-designed ivory handled knife had its own velvet case and was treated with great care. He entrusted the "sterilization" of that instrument to no one but himself. Since the number of instruments was so limited, the surgeon's expertise was not measured by the number of instruments in his black bag or case.

The biggest change in surgical instruments came about after the development of stainless steel. Today's surgeons have a vast array of instruments primarily made from stainless steel, which is composed of compounds containing carbon, chromium, iron, and other metals. This combination of compounds enables the stainless steel instrument to be more resistant to staining and corrosion but is not actually "stainless." Some other substances used are nickel, silver, and magnesium. Instruments are made of combinations of materials to aid in lengthening the life of an instrument that is subjected to repeated sterilization.

Carbon is one of the additions to stainless steel that gives surgical instruments some of their most unique properties. Stainless steel containing a higher percentage of carbon gives the instrument greater hardening but causes it to be less stain resistant. Scissors are usually made in this manner to maintain their sharpness and sharpening capabilities longer, but they are prone to staining.

The finish of an instrument is often indicative of its use. A bright finish is highly polished, reflects light, and can cause glare from the operating room lighting, which could obstruct the surgeon's vision. The dull or satin finish is less reflective with less glare and is beneficial for cardiovascular instruments. The anodized or black dull finish is preferable for use with lasers. The instruments can be ebonized by coating them with a special black chromium. The nonreflective finish is necessary to prevent accidental deflection of the laser beam from shiny instruments to an alternate site.

A final finishing process for the instrument includes inspection, surface sealing, and hand polishing.

Functions of Surgical Instruments

If correct descriptive terminology is used for the functioning parts of instruments, then no problem should exist in communicating instrument needs and demonstrating proper care of instrument techniques to others. Instruments have four basic functions in reference to their use on tissues: cutting, clamping, grasping, and retracting.

A cutting instrument such as a knife, commonly called a scalpel, is a handle on which a sharp, sterile, disposable blade is placed. The blades are designed in various shapes, such as with a rounded or a pointed tip, and are removed following the procedure. There are one-piece cutting instruments that must be sharpened, such as orthopedic osteotomes. A rounded handle with a screw to lock a disposable blade in place is a Beaver handle. The knife handles and blades are numbered so that specific blades will fit specific handles.

Scissors come in a wide variety of lengths, with curved or straight blades, with rounded or sharp tips, and with a heavy or delicate design. The choice of a scissors is usually based on the tissue or suture on which it is to be used. The handles are composed of the shank and finger rings, and the hinge area of the scissors normally contains a fitted screw. The two most common types of scissors are a Mayo scissors, which is a curved or straight, heavy blade scissors with a rounded tip, and a Metzenbaum scissors, which is a lighter, thinner, more delicate scissors with curved or straight blades (see Fig. 2–2).

Clamping instruments have a shank and finger rings as well as jaws and a box lock. For a clamping instrument to come together, the two instrument components are fitted together with a concealed pin. This hinge pin is the box lock of the instrument. It allows free movement of the two components but does not allow the parts to become disengaged.

Clamping instruments have a variety of clamping surfaces known as jaws. There are many designs of clamping jaws, and each design results in a specialized function and a special name for that particular clamp. The jaws are in contact with tissues and may have serrations that are longitudinal or transverse. The jaws are straight or curved and come in various shapes and lengths. A clamping instrument with a "tooth" at the jaw tip is a Kocher or Ochsner clamp (see Fig. 2–20). A Péan clamp is a large curved clamp with horizontal serrations extending the length of the jaw. At the base of the shank and above the finger rings are angled grooves that come together and lock the jaws in place (see Fig. 2–28). This is the rachet, and unlocking is accomplished with a slight up-and-down motion with fingers in the finger rings.

Forceps are clamping and grasping instruments. These instruments are used for temporary holding of tissue during a procedure. Forceps are designed to be held with one hand and have a flattened spring handle that is held closed by thumb and finger pressure; thus they are often referred to as thumb forceps. These instruments come in a variety of sizes and grasping points that have a grasper (tooth) or only a row of serrations for the grasping point (see Figs. 2–13 and 2–15). Thumb forceps do not have a locking mechanism, but there is another category of grasping instruments similar to a clamp with a rachet for locking. An example of this is an Allis forceps (see Fig. 2–19).

Retracting instruments are also known as exposing instruments. Retractors are used to hold back the tissue after the incision is made so that the surgeon will have a clear field of view to complete the procedure. Retracting instruments come in a variety of designs: from those with sharp to curved edges, to a thin, almost microscopic curved wire, to a wide flat or curved metal to conform to various tissue areas of depth. All are designed to hold back the tissue at a particular depth and to provide protection for vital structures during the operation. Hand-held retractors are often used in pairs (see Fig. 2–31). Retractors have a variety of handles — from those that conform to an assistant's hand to self-retaining or lighted adjustable retractors with handpiece attachments to fit on the operating room bed.

Accessory items are used to perform necessary functions during the operative procedure. Body fluids are carried away from the operative site by various tubular suctioning instruments attached to sterile tubing and connected to a vacuum system. Another example of an accessory item is a ruler that is used for accurate measuring in plastic reconstruction and orthopedic procedures (see Fig. 2–54).

Needle holders are a very important accessory instrument. Needle holders normally have a very short jaw with serrations that hold the needle attached to suture material tightly in the jaws similar to a clamping instrument. A Mayo-Hegar needle holder is one of the most common devices and comes in a variety of lengths (see Fig. 2–51). A feature of some needle holders that allows them to be repaired easily is that the jaws have a tungsten carbide inset that can be replaced when wear occurs and allows the needle to rotate instead of being held firm in the jaws of the needle holder.

CARE OF INSTRUMENTS

Since instrument costs are an important budgetary item, it is imperative that an instrument be used for that purpose for which it was designed. This will prevent costly repairs and replacement. Care and handling of instruments as they are used will also prevent damage to instruments. The process of instrument care (1) begins with the cleaning process when following their use heavier items are placed on the bottom of the decontamination basin and lighter, delicate instruments are placed on top; (2) continues with inspection of the instrument for alignment of the grasping jaws; and (3) progresses to specialized methods of preparation for sterilization and reuse.

Cleaning

All instruments when obtained from the manufacturer should be exposed to a cleaning process before they are used. If the instrument was improperly finished, the manufacturer can be contacted and asked to replace the instrument before it is used in a procedure. An instrument is designed for a specific use, and if it is used appropriately on the tissue for which it was designed, the life of the instrument will be prolonged and one can attain the expected performance from that instrument.

If all surgical instruments were treated as if they were very fine china, then our surgical instrument replacement costs would be minimized. Proper cleaning and care of instruments from point of use to terminal disinfection can be vital to the efficiency of a surgical instrument.

Point of use cleaning can be wiping the instrument free of debris with a damp or dry sponge used solely for that purpose during a surgical procedure. This gives the surgeon a clean instrument to use and prevents debris (e.g., saline, blood, protein residue) from drying on the instrument. In the operating room this technique can become an automatic response if it is practiced daily.

The flow chart in Figure 1–1 is a quick reference to the instrument care process. It can be used as a guide from the initial decontamination soak in the operating room to the choice of sterilization method for a particular instrument.

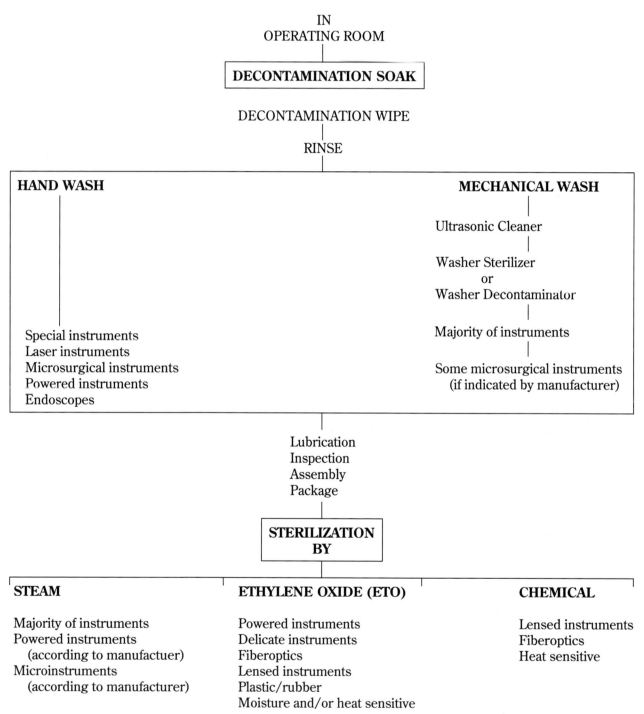

Figure 1–1. Instrument care process. (Adapted with permission from Atlas of Surgical Instrument Care. Chicago, V. Mueller Division, Baxter Healthcare Corporation, 1990.)

The cleaning process begins with a specific chemical decontamination soak process commonly used throughout the country in compliance with the Centers for Disease Control's "Recommendations for Universal Precautions" and the protection of all health care workers. This chemical decontamination is accomplished by placing the unlocked contaminated instruments in a basin of water containing the commercially available chemical decontaminant for the length of time recommended by the particular manufacturer. There are some power instruments that should not be immersed but can be wiped clean with the decontaminating solution according to the manufacturer's recommendations.

Following the decontamination process, a rinse is necessary and one of the following two processes should be followed: hand washing or mechanical washing.

Hand Washing

Washing instruments by hand with a mild, low-sudsing, neutral pH (6–8.5), warm soap solution and a soft brush is recommended for delicate microsurgical instruments and lensed instruments. An altered pH soap solution (either too alkaline or too acid) will cause staining or pitting of instruments. Steel-wool pads or abrasive powders should not be used on these instruments. The brush should be used with the instruments submerged in the cleaning solution to prevent airborne dissemination of microscopic particles during this cleaning process.

Instruments must be rinsed with distilled or demineralized water and then dried with a lint-free cloth or hot air flow. The use of distilled water rather than saline for cleaning or rinsing instruments can add years to the life of a surgical instrument by preventing the buildup of mineral residue.

A special category of instruments for which hand washing is recommended is the blackened laser instruments. These instruments must be handled carefully to prevent rubbing the blackened surfaces together and causing scratching and pitting of the silicone or black chrome finish. Endoscopy instruments and telescopes also require special hand washing and processing. Most microsurgical instruments will be hand washed but can be mechanically washed if recommended by the manufacturer.

The preparation for hand washing or mechanical washing is a time for inspection of instruments and forcing distilled water through hollow tubular (lumen) items as well as opening all closed instruments for cleaning and attesting to their proper working condition prior to sterilization and use for another patient.

Mechanical Washing

Mechanical washing can be accomplished through the use of a washer-sterilizer, a washer-decontaminator, and/or an ultrasonic washer. The manufacturer's directions should be followed in the use of commercial mechanical washers. Water temperatures and cycle times will be specific according to the manufacturer. An ultrasonic cleaning unit uses ultrasound waves through the cleaning solution to cause tiny air bubbles on the instrument surface that implode (burst inward and create a vacuum) and cause soil to disengage in a process called "cavitation." The instruments are rinsed under pressure and dried at a high temperature. Ultrasonic cleaning is very effective for removal of debris. A washer-sterilizer uses a solution agitation bath with forced air and ends with a sterilization cycle of steam under pressure. A washer-decontamination unit uses a solution agitation bath with forced air without the steam under pressure sterilization cycle. Both units clean, decontaminate, and remove excessive debris from instruments.

This mechanical washing process also begins with the timed presoak decontamination process and should be implemented prior to ultrasonic processing or washer-sterilization procedure for all instruments. It is important that pharmacologic agents such as antibacterial irrigating solutions not be allowed to remain on instruments following use.

Proper separation and loading of instruments such as heavier instruments on the bottom of the mesh basket rather than on the top of delicate instruments should occur at this time. Proper preparation should include instrumentation sorting by metals, which prevents ion transfer and pitting in some instrument finishes during the machine ultrasonic cleaning.

Powered surgical tools, special plated instruments, lensed instruments, and microscopic instruments should not be processed through a regular ultrasonic cycle.

Lubrication of instruments with an instrument bath of water-soluble, antimicrobial "milk" following each cleaning process will appropriately lubricate and protect the instrument. The instruments should not be wiped dry or rinsed following this application. A special lubricant is available for power tools per recommendation of manufacturer.

Inspection and Correction

Following the decontamination and washing, the inspection process can take place. This process of inspection for broken tips, poor alignment, corrosion, and bent instruments is essential to allow proper utilization and performance of instruments as expected. If the instrument does not function as designed, then it should be replaced. Many instruments can also be repaired by the original manufacturer.

Preparation

When an instrument is prepared for sterilization, delicate instrument tips should be protected with caps, specially designed holding mats, or foam. Ringed instruments should be placed on a rack, stringer, or pin to maintain the open position of the instrument during sterilization. Sharp points should not touch each other and need to be protected. It is important that instruments are placed in a mesh container for the free circulation of air and sterilizing agent. A towel may be used if necessary to separate and protect instruments when sterilizing an instrument set. The Association of Operating Room Nurses has issued "Standards" for size and weight of instrument sets for proper sterilization. These standards should be followed for wrapping materials, rigid containers, proper wrapping techniques, and labeling and monitoring of sterilized instruments.

Sterilization

Sterilization of instruments is accomplished with any conventionally accepted method, such as steam autoclaving, ethylene oxide exposure, and chemical immersion. The method chosen for sterilization depends on the instrument chosen and its ability to withstand heat or pressure without damaging the instrument and yet ensure sterility of the instrument. For example, an appropriate method of sterilization for a telescope would be ethylene oxide exposure since the delicate scope would be damaged by the heat and pressure of the steam sterilizer. Manufacturers of sterilizers (steam prevacuum, gravity displacement, ethylene oxide) are very specific in their instructions of operating times in reference to temperature settings, dry cycle times, and aeration cycles. Sterilizers are preset with automatic timing and locking devices to prevent human error and ensure sterilization quality control and operator safety in repeated usage.

The length of the sterilizing cycle and the delicateness of the instrument will also influence the method of sterilization. The time factor is a concern when instruments must be resterilized quickly for repeated usage in case after case each day. With much repetition of use, cleaning, and sterilization, the availability of multiple instrument sets becomes a high priority.

The flash sterilizer is normally available to an operating room but is a 3-minute, 270°, and 27-psi gravity displacement sterilizing process intended to be used in an emergency situation only, such as for a dropped item. The item or items could be sterilized quickly (flashed) to be returned to the sterile instrument area in an unwrapped sterile wire basket.

Biological indicators, chemical indicators, and mechanical monitors are all essential monitoring devices that must be integrated on a specific schedule to ensure instrument sterility. Biological monitoring is done with commercially prepared dry spores of *Bacillus stearothermophilis* (for steam sterilizers) and *Bacillus subtilis* (for ethylene oxide and dry heat sterilizers). Biological monitoring is the most reliable evaluation process for monitoring the effectiveness of the sterilizer to ensure the sterility of surgical instruments.

Manufacturers of sterilizers have specific instructions for proper sterilization, taking into consideration all the factors that must be calculated into the operation of the sterilizer or the manufacturer's recommendations for use of chemical aeration or soaking agents. Proper cleaning of the sterilizer is also a safeguard to proper care of instruments. It will aid in preventing the staining from microscopic mineral deposits.

Manufacturers recommendations of care for specific sterilizers should be followed.

Bibliography

Association for the Advancement of Medical Instrumentation: Good hospital practice: Steam sterilization and sterility assurance. In AAMI Standards and Recommended Practices, Vol 2, Sterilization. Arlington, VA, Association for the Advancement of Medical Instrumentation, 1990.

Association of Operating Room Nurses: AORN Standards and Recommended Practices for Perioperative Nursing. Denver, Association of Operating Room Nurses, 1991.

Association of Operating Room Nurses: Recommended Practices for Steam and Ethylene Oxide Sterilization. Denver, Association of Operating Room Nurses, January 1992, pp 228–240.

Atkinson, LJ, Kohn ML: Introduction to Operating Room Technique, 6th ed. New York, McGraw-Hill Book Company, 1986.

Atlas of Surgical Instrument Care. Chicago, V. Mueller Division, Baxter Healthcare Corporation, 1990.

Centers for Disease Control: Recommendations for preventing transmission of human immunodeficiency virus and hepatitis B virus to patients during exposure-prone invasive procedures. MMWR 40:RR8, July 12, 1991.

Centers for Disease Control: Recommendations for prevention of HIV transmission in health care settings. MMWR 36:6S, 1987.

Fuller JR: Surgical Technology Principles and Practice, 2nd ed. Philadelphia, W.B. Saunders, 1986.

General Instrumentation Atlas, vol 1. Chicago, V. Mueller Division, Baxter Healthcare Corporation, 1987.

Groah LK: Operating Room Nursing: Perioperative Practice, 2nd ed. East Norwalk, CT, Appleton & Lange, 1990.

Meeker MH, Rothrock JC: Alexander's Care of the Patient in Surgery, 9th ed. C.V. Mosby–Year Book Medical Publishers, St. Louis, 1991.

Miltex Surgical Instruments. Lake Success, NY. Miltex Instrument Company, 1986.

Surgical Armamentarium. Chicago, V. Mueller Division, Baxter Healthcare Corporation, 1989.

CHAPTER

2

Basic Functions

Cutting Instruments

Scalpel Handles and Blades

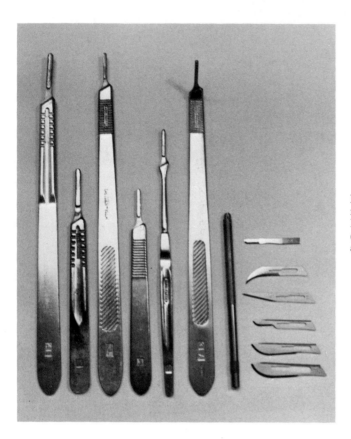

Figure 2–1. Scalpel handles *(left to right):* No. 4 long, No. 4 regular, No. 3 long, No. 3 regular, No. 7, and No. 3 angled. Beaver chuck handle for Beaver blades. Disposable blades *(top to bottom):* No. 64 Beaver, No. 12, No. 11, No. 15, No. 10, and No. 20.

Scissors

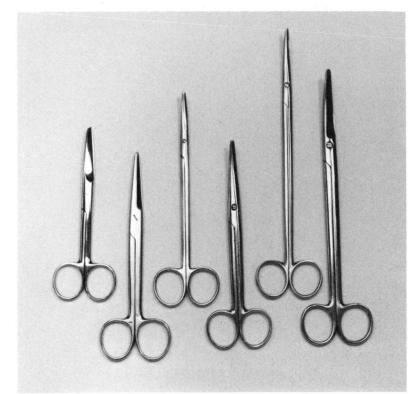

Figure 2–2. *Left to right.* Suture scissors, straight Mayo scissors, Metzenbaum scissors, curved Mayo scissors, long Metzenbaum scissors, and long Mayo scissors.

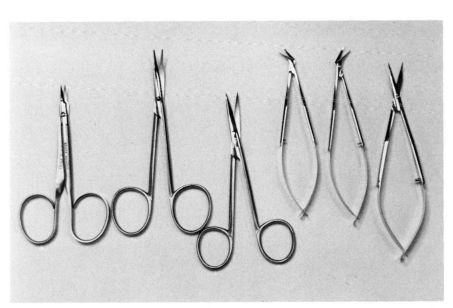

Figure 2–3. *Left to right.* Stitch scissors, Stevens tenotomy scissors, Stevens iris scissors, left and right corneal scissors, and Wescott scissors.

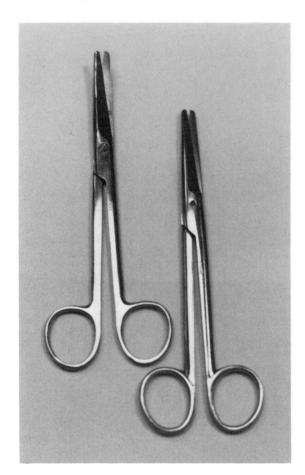

Figure 2–4. *Left.* Mayo curved scissors. *Right.* Mayo straight scissors.

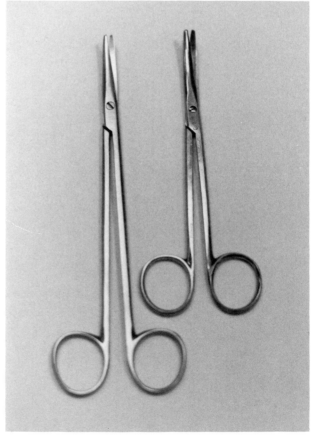

Figure 2–5. *Left.* Regular Metzenbaum scissors. *Right.* Short Metzenbaum scissors.

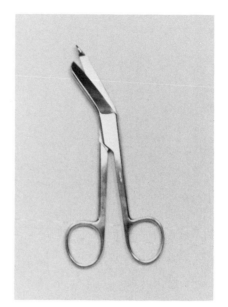

Figure 2–6. Bandage scissors.

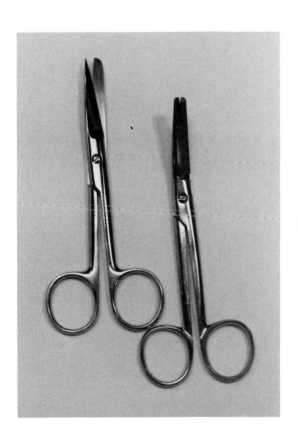

Figure 2–7. *Left.* Straight suture scissors. *Right.* Angled suture scissors.

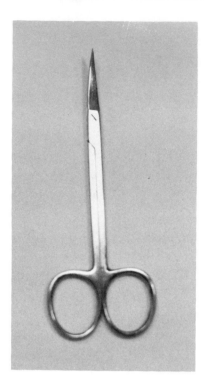

Figure 2–8. Iris scissors.

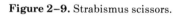

Figure 2–9. Strabismus scissors.

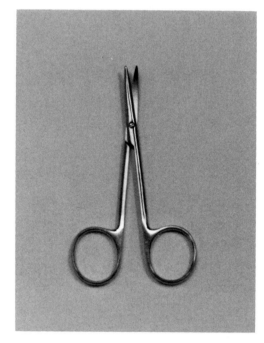

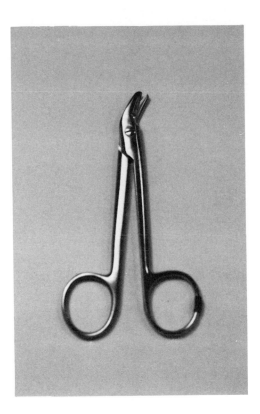

Figure 2–10. Wire-cutting scissors.

Figure 2–11. Potts-Smith scissors.

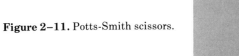

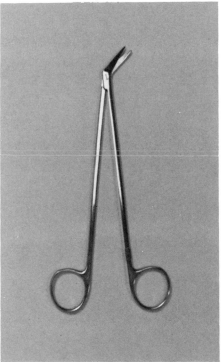

Tissue Forceps

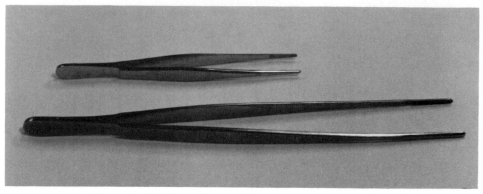

Figure 2–12. Tissue forceps without teeth: long and regular.

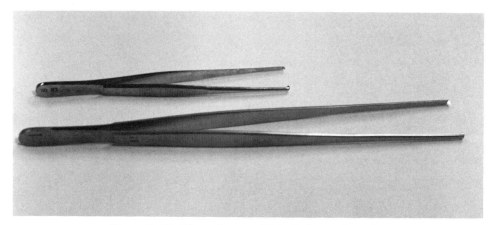

Figure 2–13. Tissue forceps with teeth: long and regular.

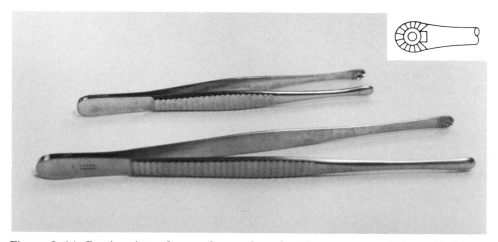

Figure 2–14. Russian tissue forceps: long and regular. (*Inset* courtesy of Baxter Healthcare Corporation.)

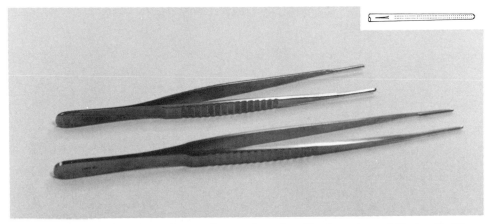

Figure 2–15. DeBakey tissue forceps: long and regular. (*Inset* courtesy of Baxter Healthcare Corporation.)

Figure 2–16. *Top to bottom.* Adson tissue forceps without teeth, Adson forceps with teeth, and Brown-Adson forceps.

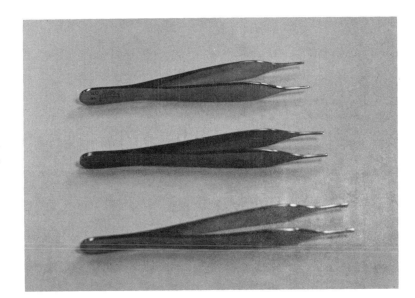

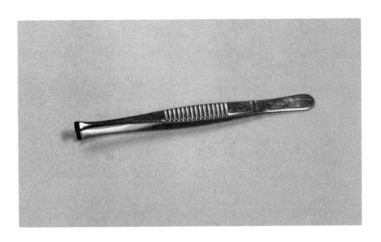

Figure 2–17. Hayes Martin forceps.

Grasping Instruments

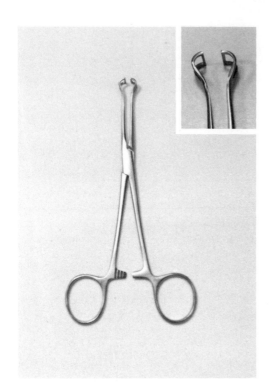

Figure 2–18. Babcock clamp.

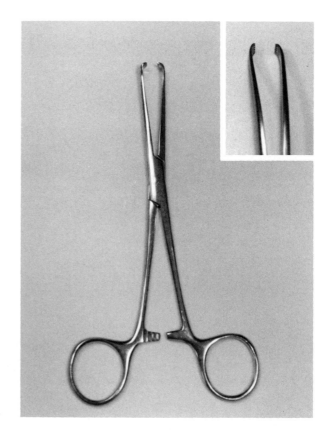

Figure 2–19. Allis clamp.

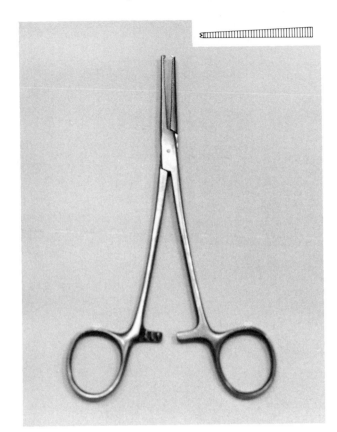

Figure 2–20. Kocher (Ochsner) clamp. (*Inset* courtesy of Baxter Healthcare Corporation.)

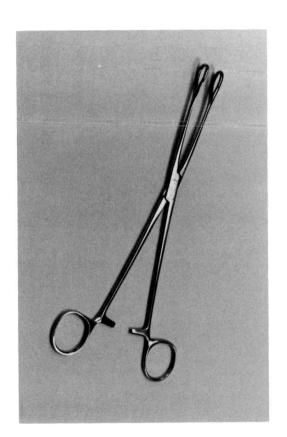

Figure 2–21. Foerster sponge forceps.

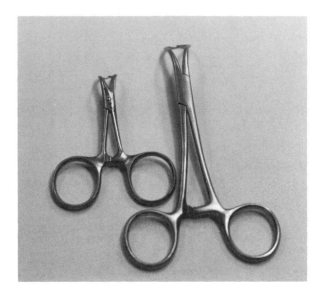

Figure 2–22. Backhaus towel clamps: large and small.

Clamping Instruments

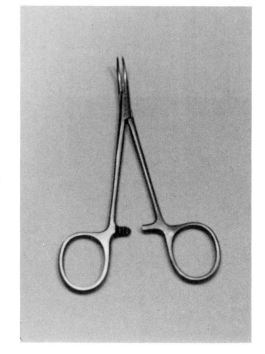

Figure 2–23. Mosquito (Halsted) clamp.

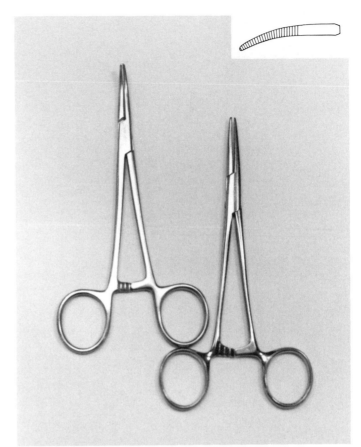

Figure 2–24. Kelly clamps: curved and straight. (*Inset* courtesy of Baxter Healthcare Corporation.)

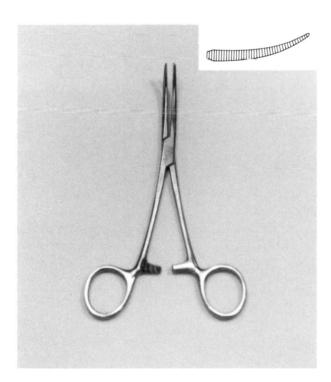

Figure 2–25. Curved Crile clamp. (*Inset* courtesy of Baxter Healthcare Corporation.)

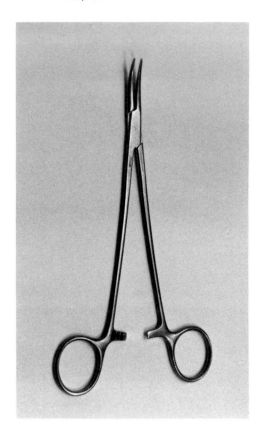

Figure 2–26. Adson hemostatic forceps.

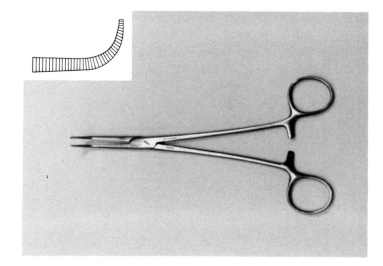

Figure 2–27. Right-angled Mixter forceps. (*Inset* courtesy of Baxter Healthcare Corporation.)

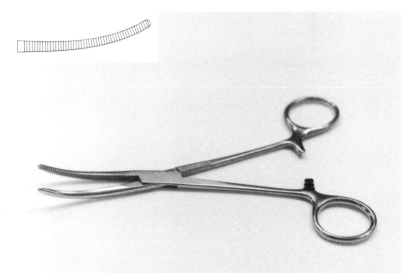

Figure 2–28. Péan (Rochester-Péan) clamp. (*Inset* courtesy of Baxter Healthcare Corporation.)

Retractors

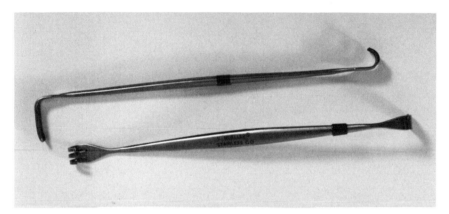

Figure 2–29. Senn retractors.

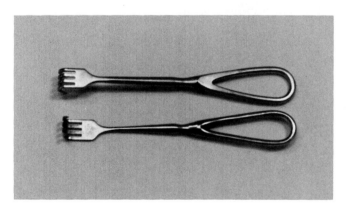

Figure 2–30. Rake (Volkmann) retractors.

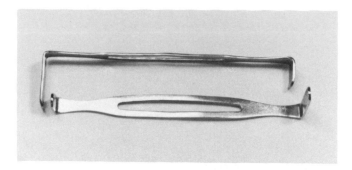

Figure 2–31. U.S. Army-Navy retractors.

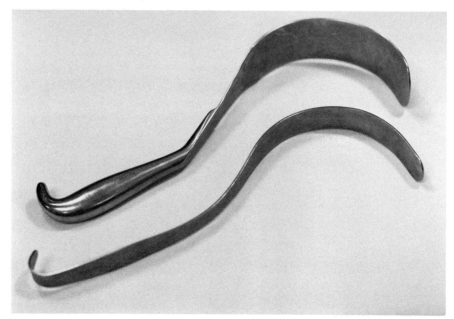

Figure 2–32. Deaver retractors.

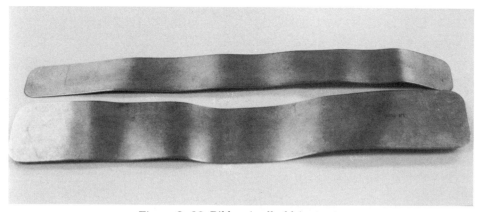

Figure 2–33. Ribbon (malleable) retractors.

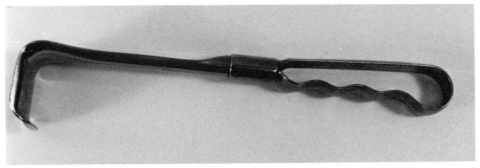

Figure 2–34. Richardson retractor.

Figure 2–35. Weitlaner retractor.

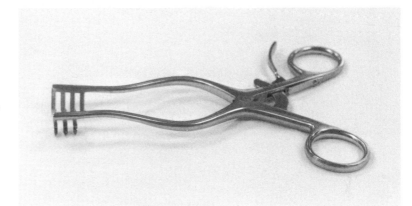

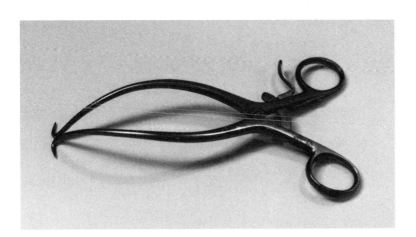

Figure 2–36. Gelpi retractor.

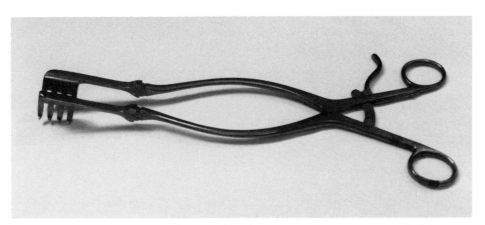

Figure 2–37. Beckman retractor.

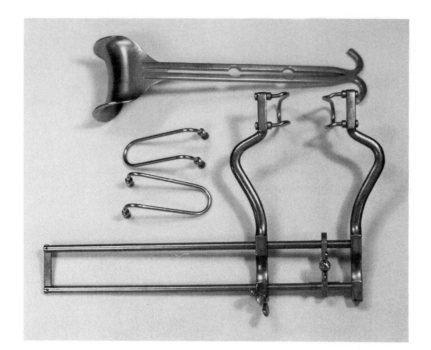

Figure 2–38. Balfour abdominal retractor, one center blade, four wire side blades.

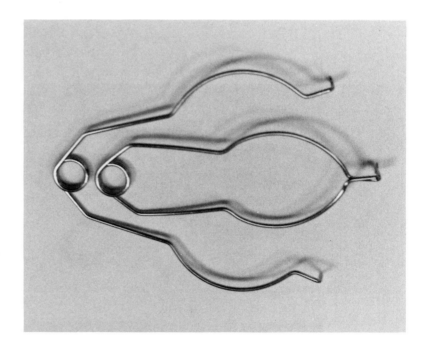

Figure 2–39. Spring wire retractors.

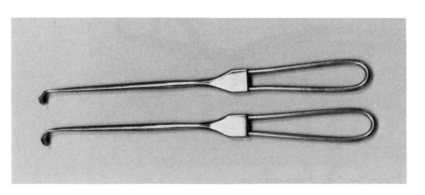

Figure 2–40. Vein retractors.

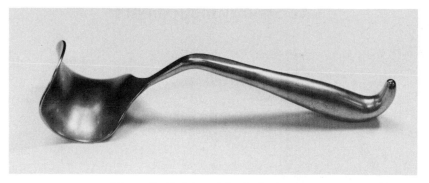

Figure 2–41. Mayo abdominal retractor.

Figure 2–42. *Top.* Crile retractors. *Bottom.* Childrens' Hospital retractors.

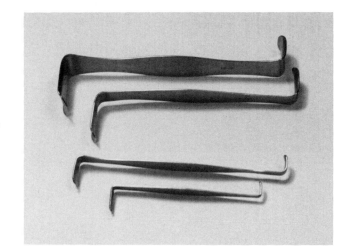

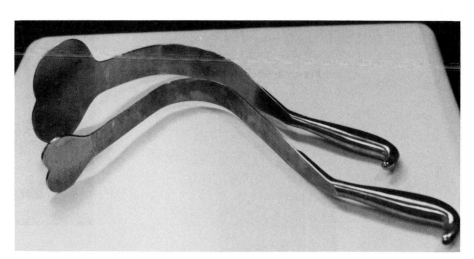

Figure 2–43. Harrington retractors.

Accessory Instruments

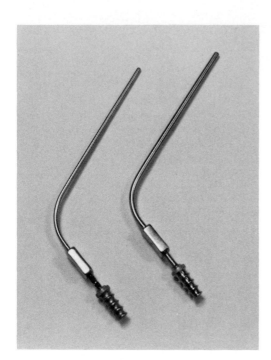

Figure 2–44. Frazier suction tips.

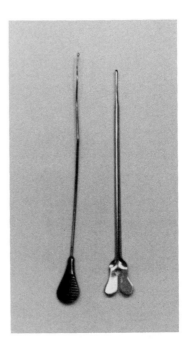

Figure 2–45. Buie probe, groove director.

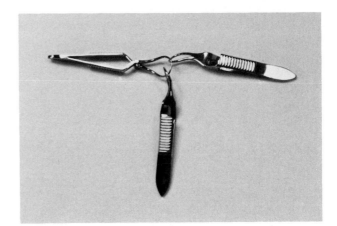

Figure 2–46. Jones towel clips.

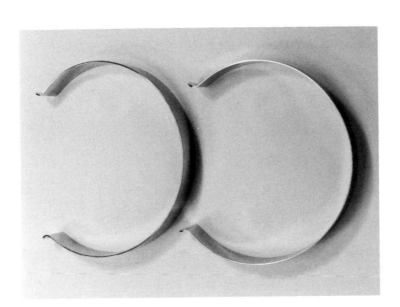

Figure 2–47. Bethea sheet holders.

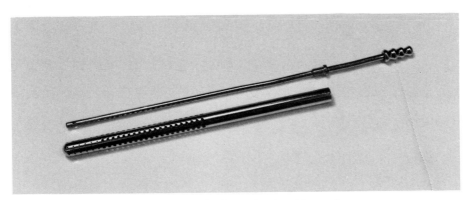

Figure 2–48. Poole suction tip with guard.

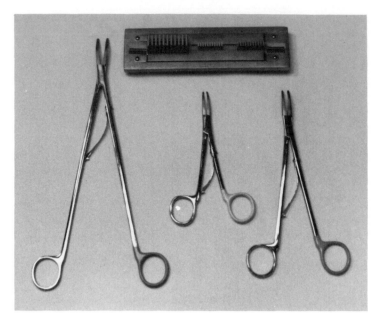

Figure 2–49. Hemoclip appliers *(left to right):* long, short, medium. *Top.* Hemoclip holder with hemoclips.

Needle Holders

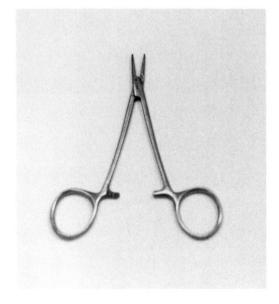

Figure 2–50. Webster needle holder.

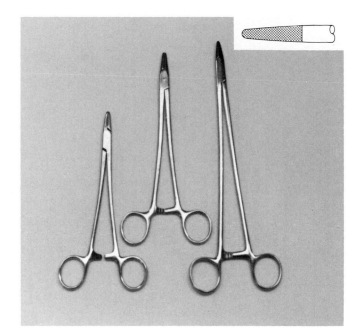

Figure 2–51. *Left to right.* Collier needle holder, long Mayo-Hegar needle holder, and extra-long Mayo-Hegar needle holder. (*Inset* courtesy of Baxter Healthcare Corporation.)

Measuring Devices

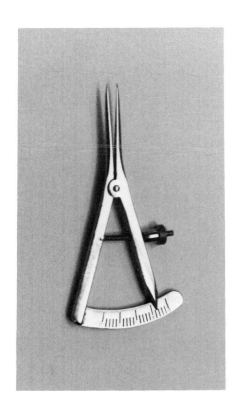

Figure 2–52. Castroviejo caliper.

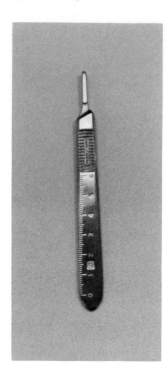

Figure 2–53. No. 3 knife handle.

Figure 2–54. Zimmer ruler.

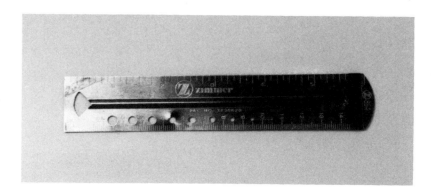

CHAPTER

3

Minor Instrument Sets

MINOR INSTRUMENT SET

The instrument set in Figure 3–1 is representative of the instruments needed for minor surgical procedures. It is impossible to determine the exact number of curved hemostats or Kocher clamps that will be needed for every minor procedure. Surgeons' preferences vary greatly, and it will always be necessary to add instruments or to take away items to keep the number of instruments to a minimum for cost effectiveness, wear and tear on instruments, and cost of washing, preparation, and sterilization. The set pictured here should only serve as a guideline on which to build a set to meet your institution's needs.

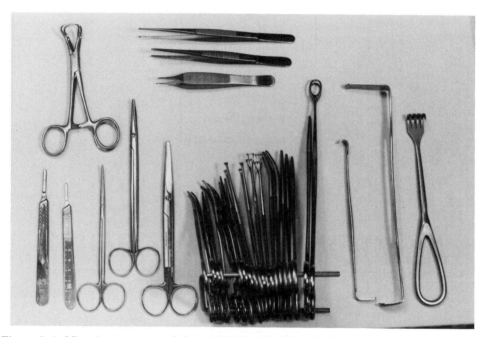

Figure 3–1. Minor instrument set *(left to right):* No. 4 Knife handle, No. 3 knife handle, small Metzenbaum scissors, regular Metzenbaum scissors, straight Mayo scissors, curved mosquito clamps, straight mosquito clamps, curved Kelly clamps, straight Kelly clamps, two Allis clamps, two Babcock clamps, two Péan clamps, two straight Kocher clamps, short needle holder, long needle holder, Foerster sponge forceps, Senn retractor, U.S. Army-Navy retractor, rake retractor. *Top.* Two towel clamps, Adson tissue forceps, tissue forceps without teeth, and tissue forceps with teeth. Retractors would be used in pairs.

Suture Set

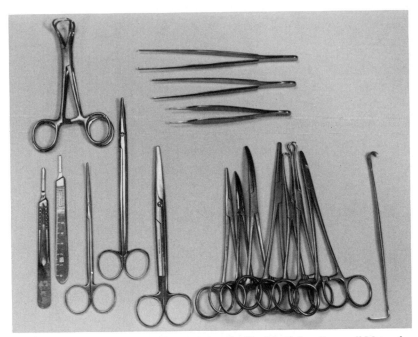

Figure 3–2. Suture set *(left to right):* No. 4 knife handle; No. 3 knife handle; small Metzenbaum scissors; regular Metzenbaum scissors; straight Mayo scissors; straight Kelly clamp; curved Crile, Péan, Kocher, Allis, and Babcock clamps; Webster needle holder; Senn retractor. *Top.* Two towel clamps, Adson tissue forceps, plain tissue forceps without teeth, and tissue forceps with teeth. Senn retractors are used in pairs. This minor suture set could be used for small procedures and instruments could be added for specific needs and size of patient.

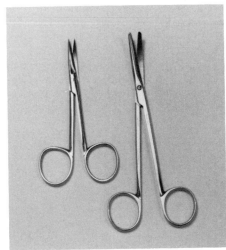

Figure 3–3. *Left.* Iris scissors. *Right.* Small Metzenbaum scissors.

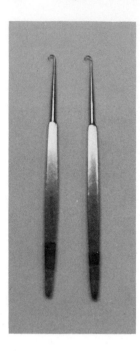

Figure 3–4. Skin hooks.

Incision and Drainage

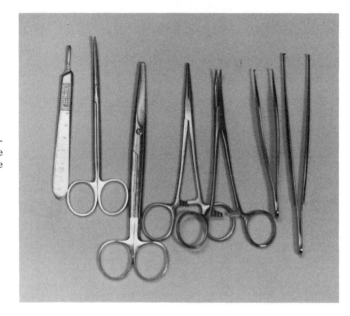

Figure 3–5. *Left to right.* No. 3 knife handle, small Metzenbaum scissors, straight Mayo scissors, straight Crile clamp, curved Kelly clamp, Adson tissue forceps, and tissue forceps with teeth.

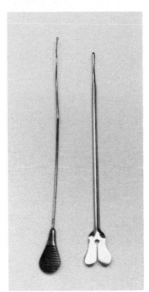

Figure 3–6. Buie probe and groove director.

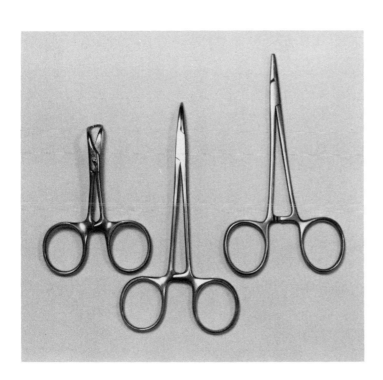

Figure 3–7. *Left to right.* Towel clip, curved Kelly clamp, and Webster needle holder.

Lesion Biopsy

Use minor instrument set and add the following:

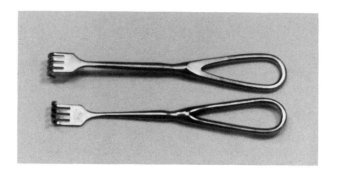

Figure 3–8. Rake retractors.

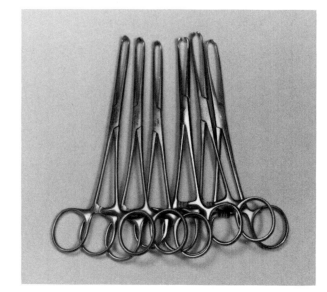

Figure 3–9. Allis clamps.

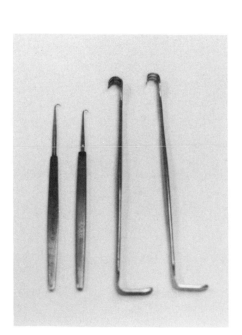

Figure 3–10. Skin hooks and Senn retractors.

Hernia Repair

Use minor instrument set and add the following:

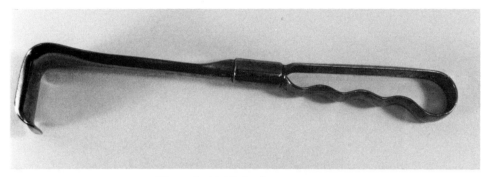

Figure 3–11. Richardson retractor.

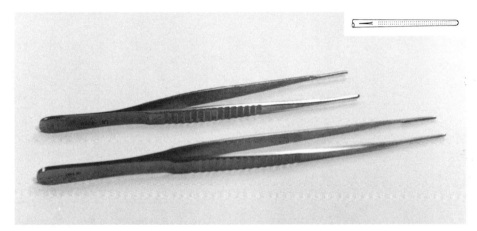

Figure 3–12. DeBakey tissue forceps: long and regular.

Figure 3–13. Right-angled Mixter forceps.

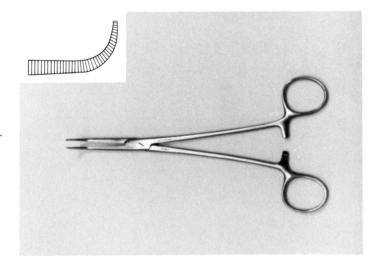

Major Instrument Sets

LAPAROTOMY

The major laparotomy set varies greatly according to geographic areas. The instruments in Figure 4–1 can be repeated in multiples according to the needs of the institution and surgeons. Many retractor choices are available and can be added or placed in a separate set. A common choice to be added is a Balfour self-retaining retractor.

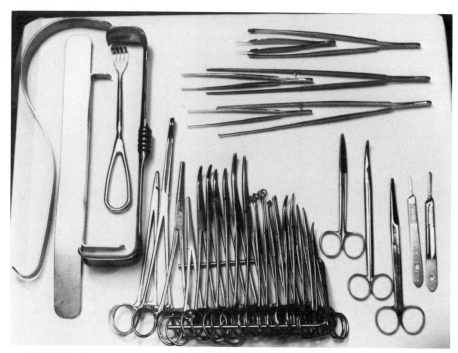

Figure 4–1. Major laparotomy set *(left to right):* Deaver, malleable, U.S. Army, rake, Richardson double-ended retractor; Mayo-Hegar needle holder, Foerster sponge forceps, straight Kocher clamp, long and short; Mixter and Adson hemostatic forceps; Péan, Babcock, Allis, curved Crile, straight Kelly, and mosquito clamps, towel clips; curved Mayo, Metzenbaum, and straight Mayo scissors; Nos. 3 and 4 knife handles. *Top right.* Tissue forceps, Adson forceps with teeth, and Russian, long and short plain forceps and long and short forceps with teeth.

Appendectomy–Exploratory Laparotomy

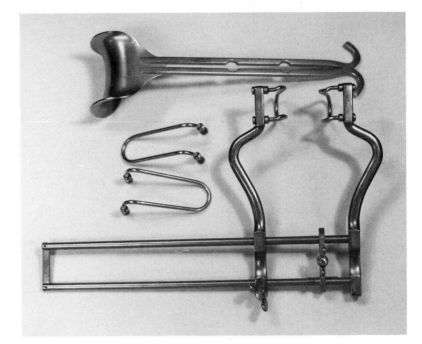

Figure 4–2. Balfour abdominal retractor, one center blade, four wire side blades.

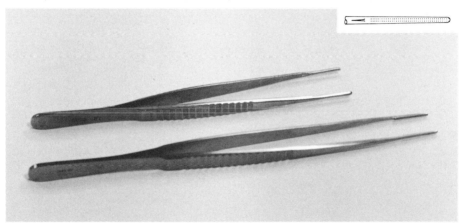

Figure 4–3. DeBakey tissue forceps: long and regular. (*Inset* courtesy of Baxter Healthcare Corporation.)

Cholecystectomy

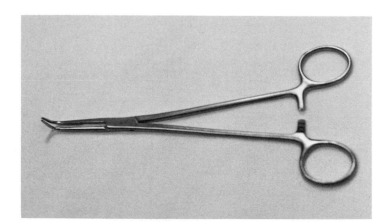

Figure 4–4. Mixter Right-angled forceps.

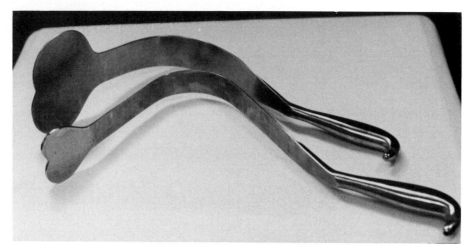

Figure 4–5. Harrington retractors.

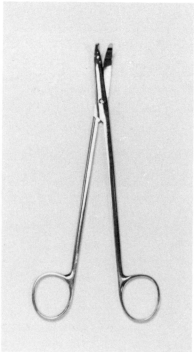

Figure 4–6. Thorek-Feldman scissors (for gallbladder surgery).

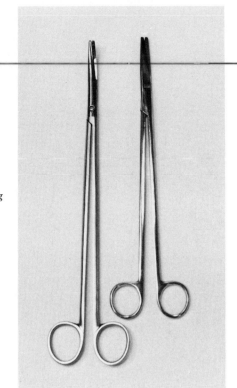

Figure 4–7. *Left.* Long Metzenbaum scissors. *Right.* Mayo-Harrington dissecting scissors.

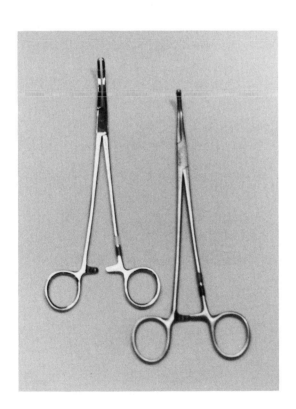

Figure 4–8. Borge cystic duct catheter clamps.

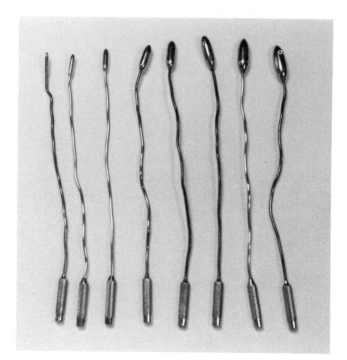

Figure 4–9. Bakes common bile duct dilators.

Figure 4–10. Ochsner (Fenger) flexible gallstone probe.

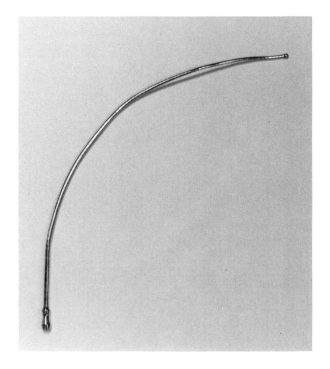

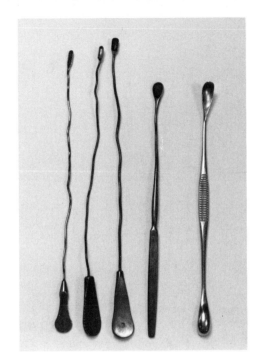

Figure 4–11. *Left to right.* Mayo cystic duct scoop, Mayo common duct scoops, Berens common duct scoop, and Ferguson double-ended gallstone scoop.

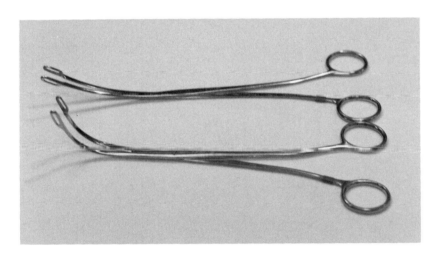

Figure 4–12. Randall stone forceps.

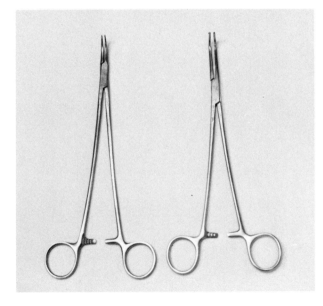

Figure 4–13. *Left.* Fine Adson hemostatic clamp. *Right.* Long fine Mixter (right-angled) forceps.

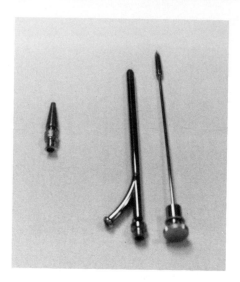

Figure 4–14. *Left to right.* Adapter, Ochsner gallbladder trocar, and stylet.

Stomach–Intestinal Procedures

Figure 4–15. Long Babcock clamp.

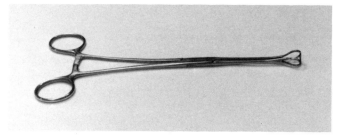

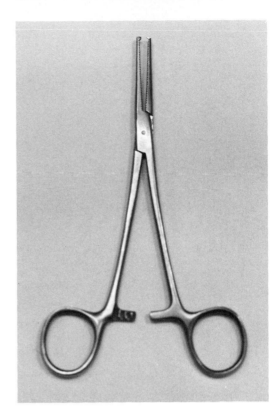

Figure 4–16. Long Kocher clamp.

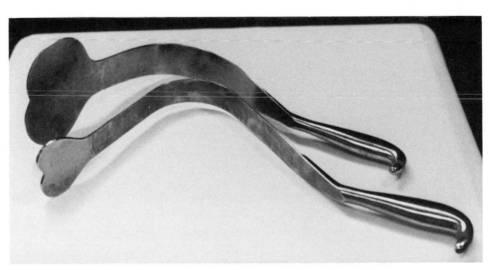

Figure 4–17. Harrington retractors.

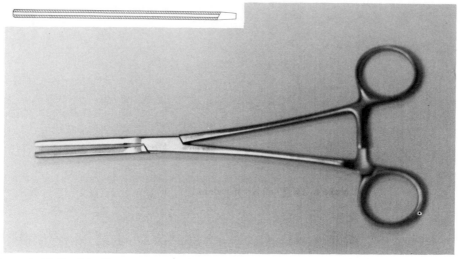

Figure 4–18. Straight Glassman noncrushing intestinal clamp. (*Inset* Courtesy of Baxter Healthcare Corporation.)

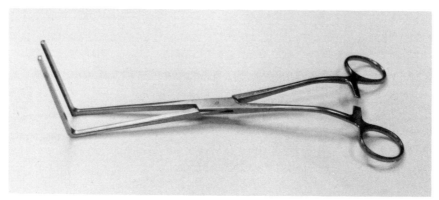

Figure 4–19. Angled Glassman intestinal clamp.

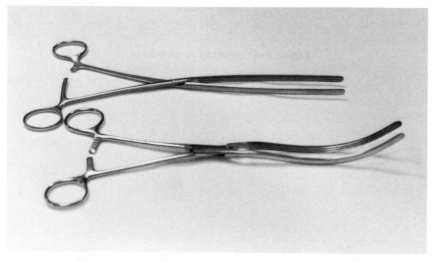

Figure 4–20. Kocher intestinal forceps: straight and curved.

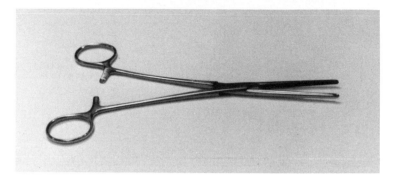

Figure 4–21. Straight Carmalt clamp.

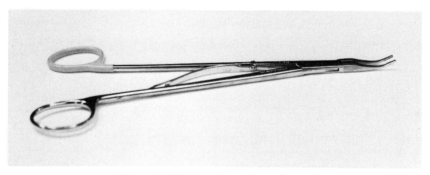

Figure 4–22. Long hemoclip applier.

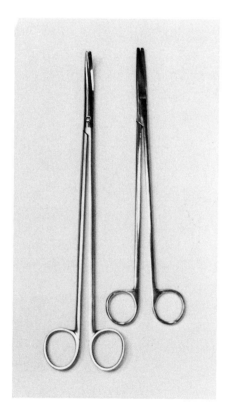

Figure 4–23. *Left.* Long Metzenbaum scissors. *Right.* Mayo-Harrington dissecting scissors.

Gynecologic Surgery

Dilatation and Curettage

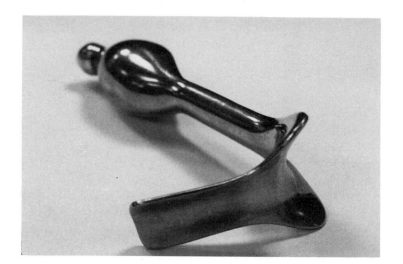

Figure 5–1. Auvard vaginal speculum.

Figure 5–2. Jackson vaginal retractor.

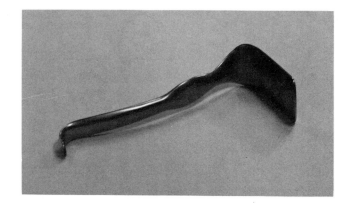

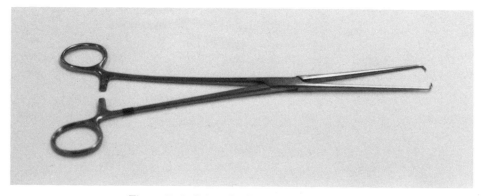

Figure 5–3. Schroeder-Braun uterine tenaculum.

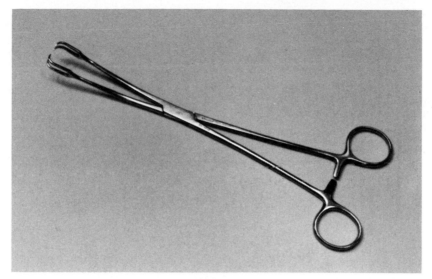

Figure 5–4. Schroeder uterine tenaculum.

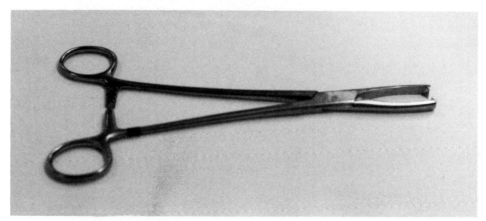

Figure 5–5. Straight Museux uterine vulsellum forceps.

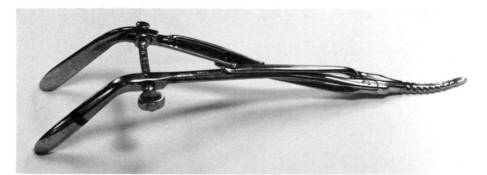

Figure 5–6. Goodell uterine dilator.

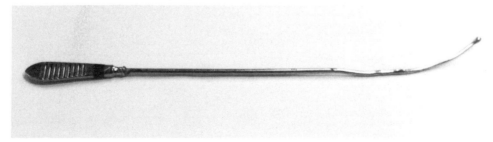

Figure 5–7. Sims uterine sound.

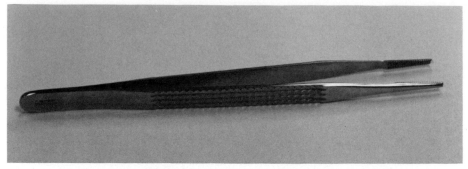

Figure 5–8. Curtis tissue forceps.

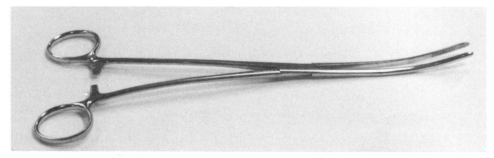

Figure 5–9. Bozeman uterine packing forceps.

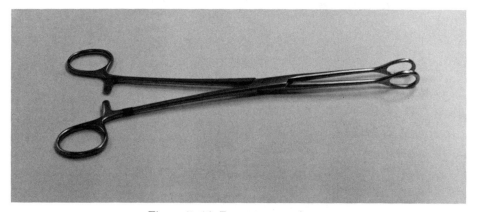

Figure 5–10. Foerster sponge forceps.

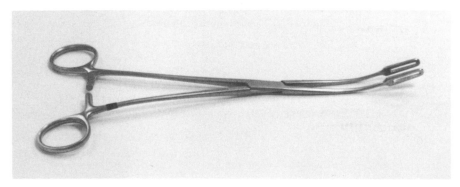

Figure 5–11. Fletcher-Van Doren uterine polyp forceps.

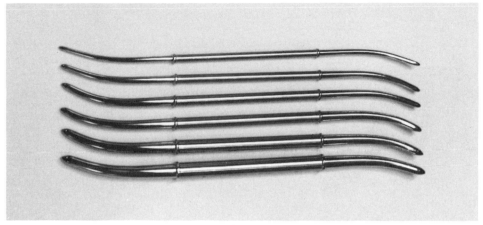

Figure 5–12. Hank uterine dilators.

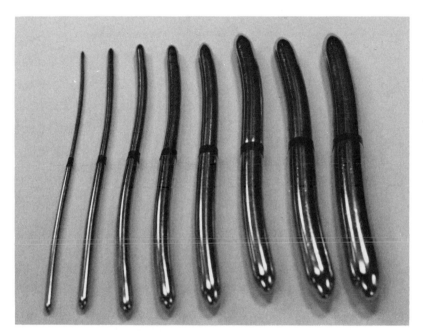

Figure 5–13. Hegar uterine dilators.

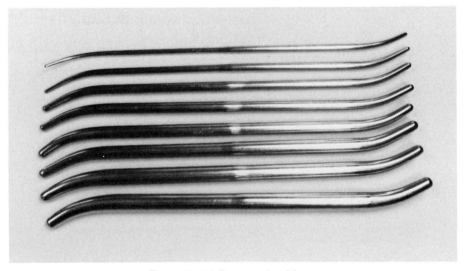

Figure 5–14. Pratt uterine dilators.

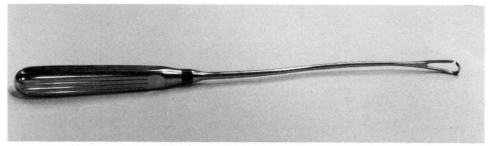

Figure 5–15. Sims sharp curette.

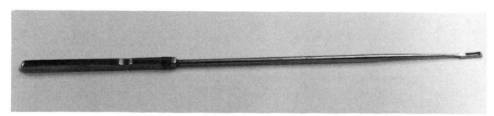

Figure 5–16. Heaney uterine curette.

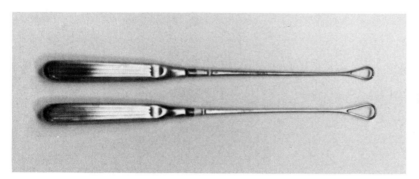

Figure 5–17. Thomas dull uterine curettes.

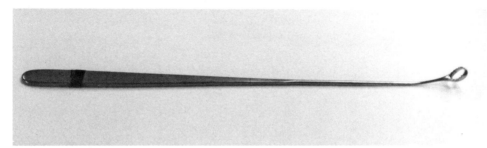

Figure 5–18. Kevorkian-Younge endocervical curette.

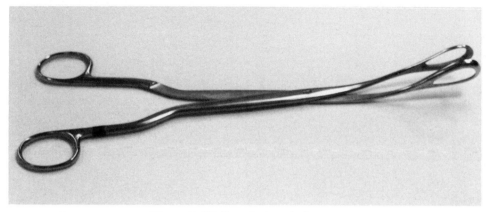

Figure 5–19. Barrett placenta forceps.

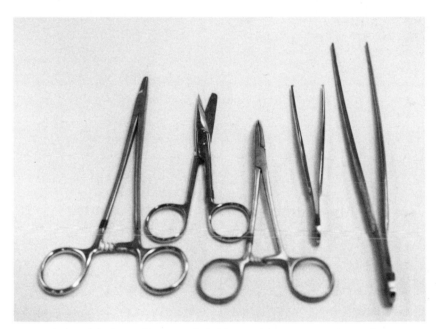

Figure 5–20. *Left to right.* Mayo-Hegar needle holder; straight operating scissors; Crile (Mayo) hemostat, short (5-inch) tissue forceps with teeth; and long (10-inch) tissue forceps without teeth.

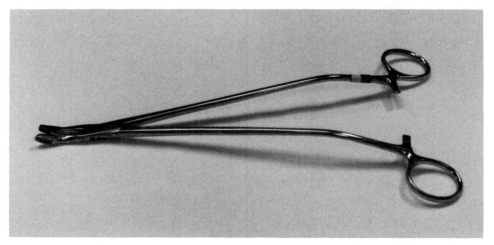

Figure 5–21. Van Doren uterine biopsy forceps.

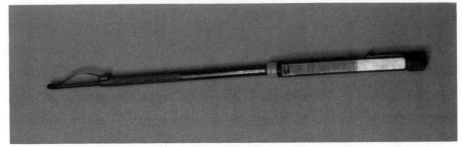

Figure 5–22. Fleming knife handle with blade attached.

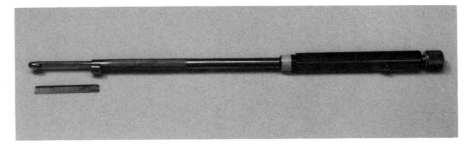

Figure 5–23. Fleming knife handle with blade.

Abdominal-Vaginal Hysterectomy

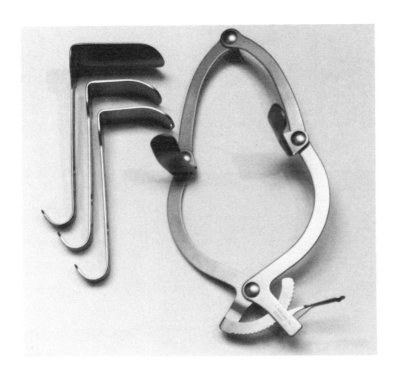

Figure 5–24. O'Sullivan-O'Connor retractor with three center blades and two side blades.

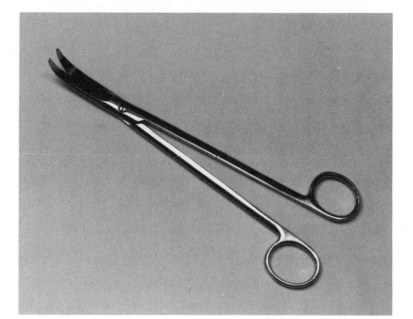

Figure 5–25. Jorgenson scissors.

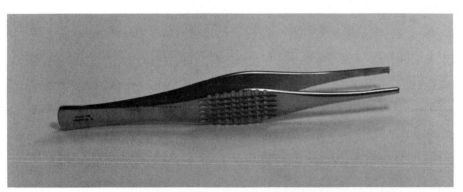

Figure 5–26. Ferris Smith tissue forceps.

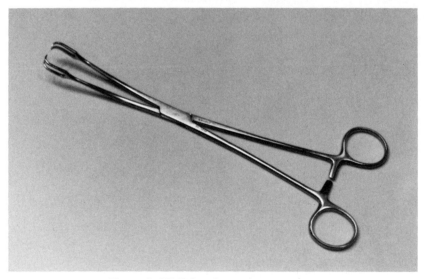

Figure 5–27. Schroeder uterine tenaculum.

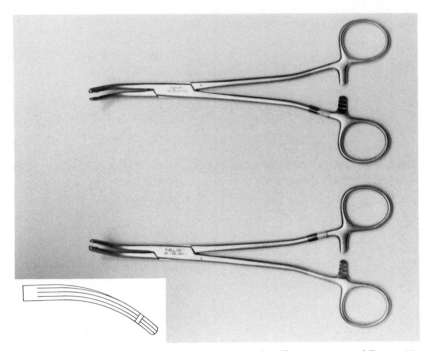

Figure 5–28. Glenner hysterectomy forceps; left and right. (*Inset* courtesy of Baxter Healthcare Corporation.)

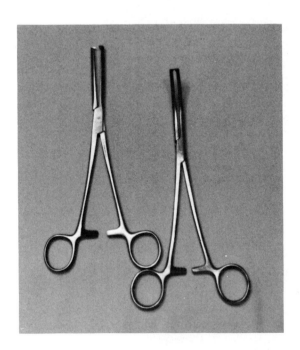

Figure 5–29. Long, straight *(left)* and curved *(right)* Kocher forceps.

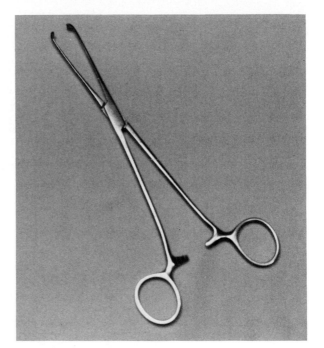

Figure 5–30. Long Allis forceps.

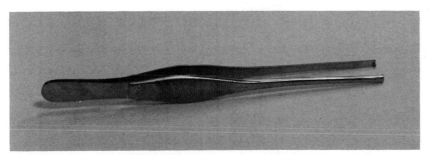

Figure 5–31. Heaney tissue forceps.

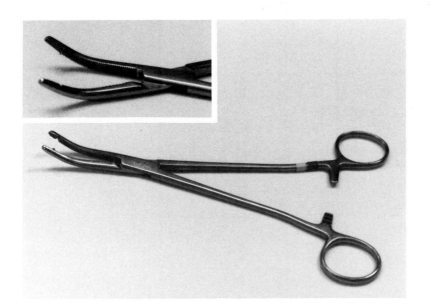

Figure 5–32. Heaney forceps.

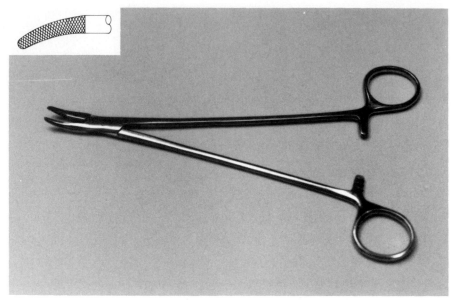

Figure 5–33. Heaney needle holder. (*Inset* courtesy of Baxter Healthcare Corporation.)

Vaginal Delivery

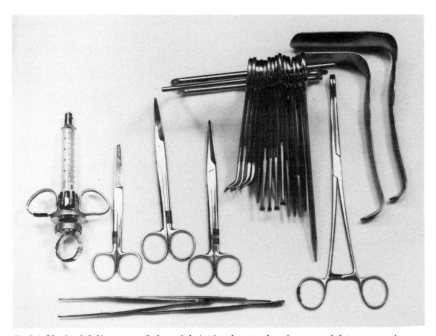

Figure 5–34. Vaginal delivery set *(left to right):* 10-ml control syringe, straight suture scissors, curved Mayo scissors, straight Mayo scissors, towel clips, straight Crile clamp, four Allis clamps, four small Kocher clamps, long needle holder, Foerster sponge forceps, and long and short Jackson retractors. *Bottom.* Tissue forceps with and without teeth.

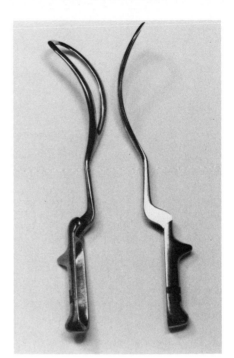

Figure 5–35. DeLee obstetrical forceps.

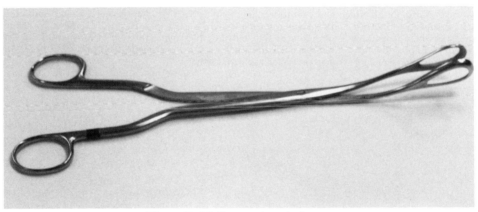

Figure 5–36. Barrett placenta forceps.

Cesarean Section

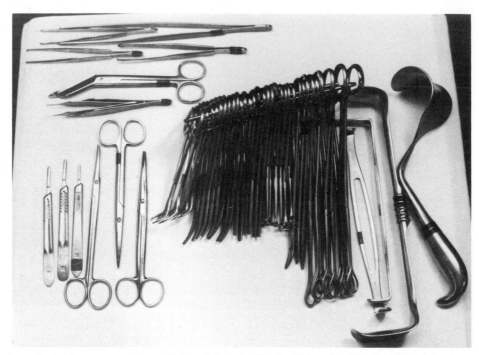

Figure 5–37. Cesarean section set *(left to right):* Two No. 4 knife handles, No. 3 handle; Metzenbaum, curved and straight Mayo scissors; four towel clips, eight curved Crile clamps, six Kocher clamps, four Allis clamps, two Babcock clamps, Heaney needle holder, two Mayo-Hegar needle holders, six sponge forceps, two U.S. Army-Navy retractors, double-ended Richardson retractor, and Mayo retractor. *Top to bottom.* Long and short tissue forceps, plain; regular tissue forceps with teeth; Russian tissue forceps; bandage scissors; and Adson tissue forceps with teeth.

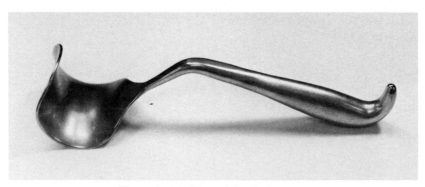

Figure 5–38. Mayo abdominal retractor.

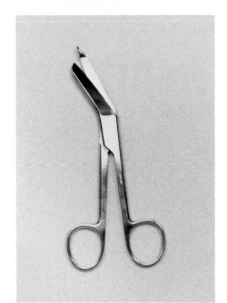

Figure 5–39. Bandage scissors.

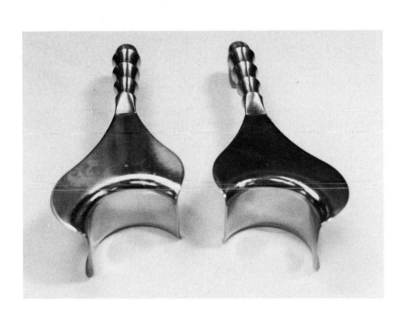

Figure 5–40. DeLee retractors, left and right.

Rectal Surgery

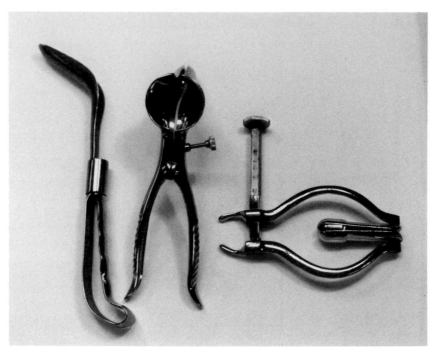

Figure 6–1. *Left to right.* Sawyer retractor, Pratt rectal speculum, Buie-Smith self-retaining anal retractor.

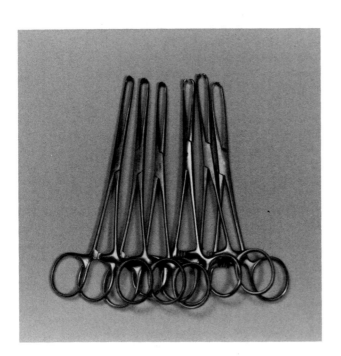

Figure 6–2. Allis clamps.

Figure 6–3. Cushing bayonet tissue forceps.

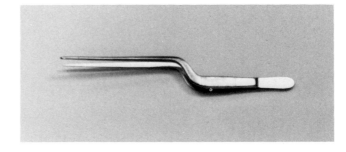

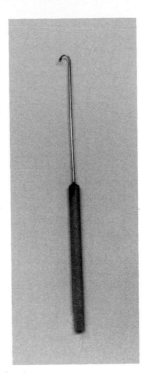

Figure 6–4. Rosser crypt hook.

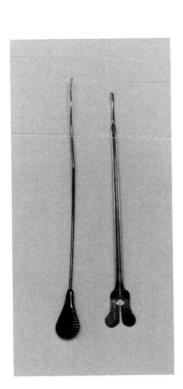

Figure 6–5. *Left.* Buie probe. *Right.* Groove director.

CHAPTER 7

Genitourinary Surgery

Genitourinary-Abdominal Procedures

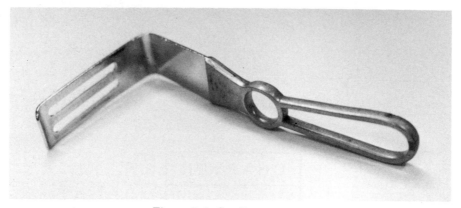

Figure 7–1. Coryllos retractor.

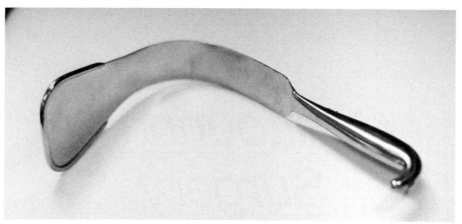

Figure 7–2. B.E. Glass abdominal retractor.

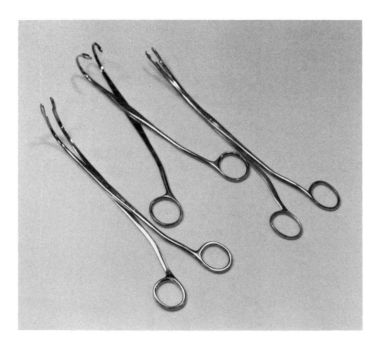

Figure 7–3. Randalll stone forceps.

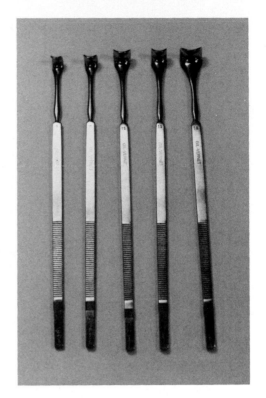

Figure 7–4. Gil-Vernet renal sinus retractors (9–18 mm).

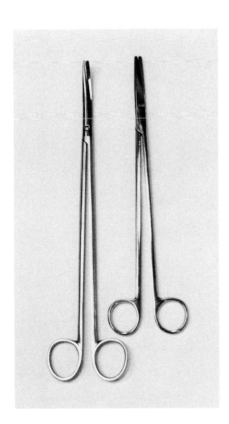

Figure 7–5. *Left.* Long Metzenbaum scissors. *Right.* Mayo-Harrington dissecting scissors.

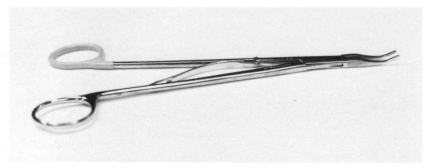

Figure 7–6. Long hemoclip applier.

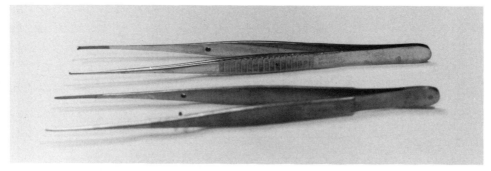

Figure 7–7. Potts-Smith tissue forceps, with and without teeth.

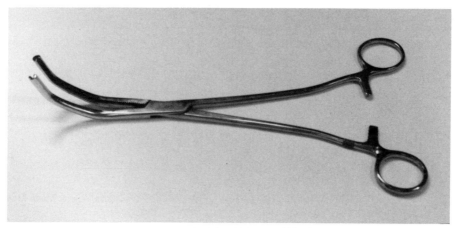

Figure 7–8. Walther kidney pedicle clamp.

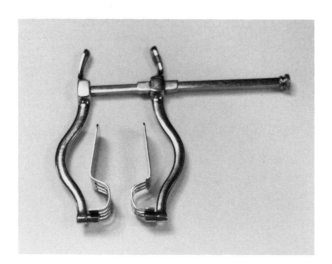

Figure 7–9. Mason-Judd bladder retractor.

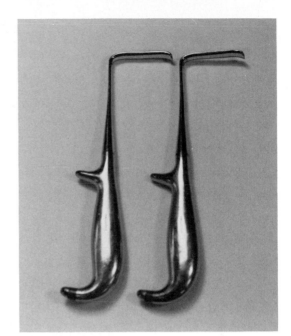

Figure 7–10. Young lateral retractors.

Circumcision

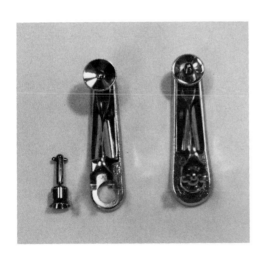

Figure 7–11. Yellen circumcision clamps.

Meatotomy

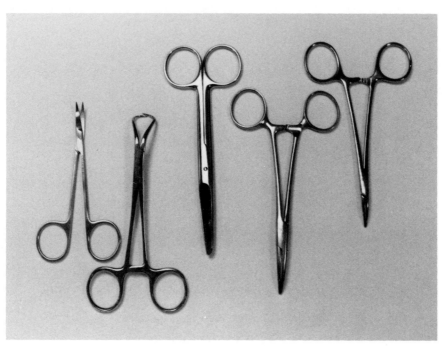

Figure 7–12. Meatotomy set *(left to right):* Curved iris scissors, Backhaus towel clamp, utility scissors, Kelly hemostat, and mosquito hemostat.

CHAPTER
8

Plastic Reconstructive Surgery

PLASTIC REPAIR

Minor instrument or suture instrument sets are used with specific additional instruments for specialty surgeons.

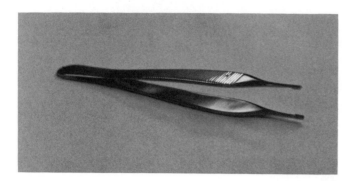

Figure 8–1. Brown-Adson tissue forceps.

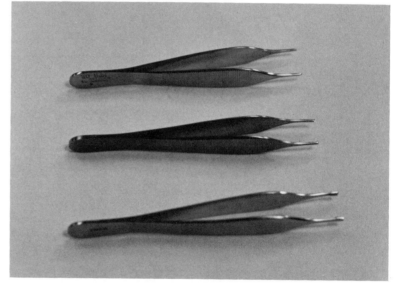

Figure 8–2. *Top to bottom.* Adson tissue forceps without teeth, Adson tissue forceps with teeth, and Brown-Adson tissue forceps.

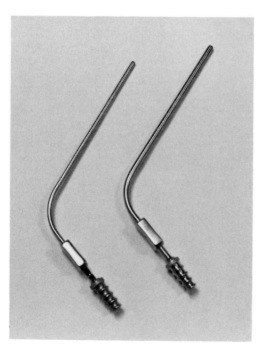

Figure 8–3. Frazier suction tips.

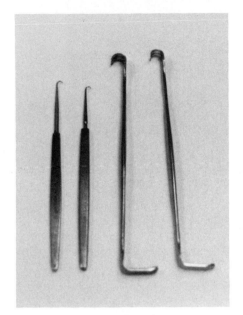

Figure 8–4. Skin hooks and Senn retractors.

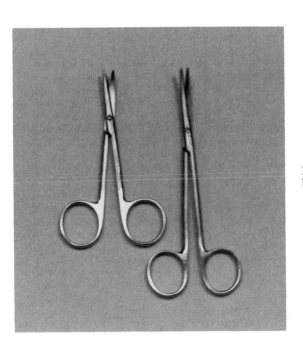

Figure 8–5. *Left.* Curved strabismus scissors. *Right.* Small Metzenbaum scissors.

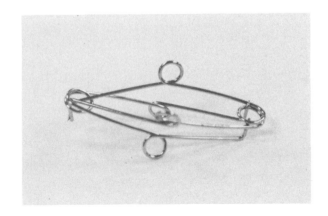

Figure 8–6. Baby spring wire retractors.

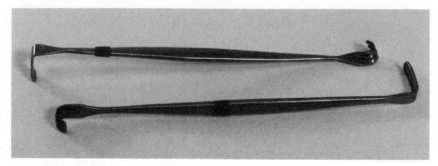

Figure 8–7. Senn retractors.

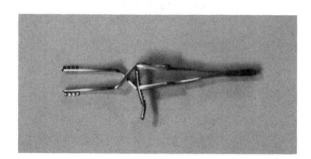

Figure 8–8. Heiss retractor.

Figure 8–9. Weitlaner retractor.

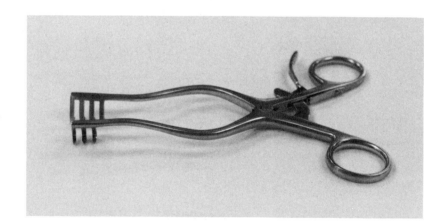

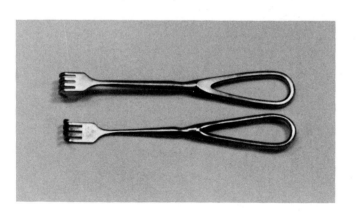

Figure 8–10. Rake (Volkmann) retractors.

Figure 8–11. Vein retractors.

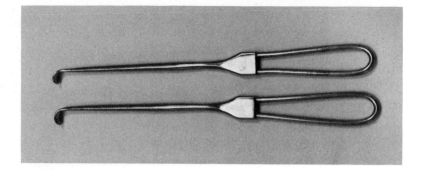

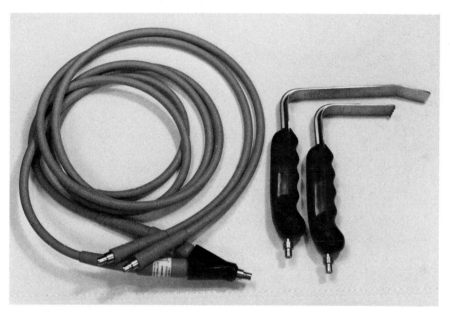

Figure 8–12. Fiberoptic lighted retractors.

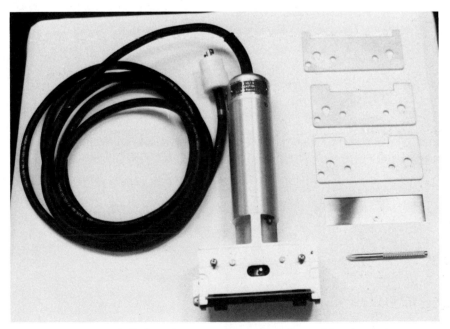

Figure 8–13. Padgett dermatome (to attach to foot pedal and power).

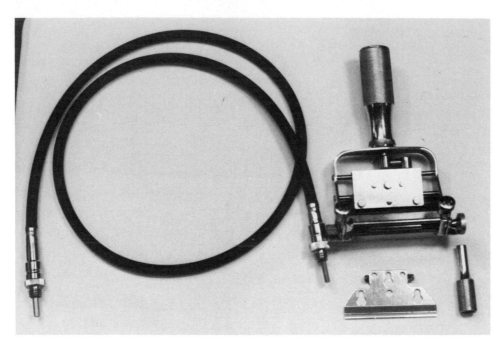

Figure 8–14. Brown dermatome (to attach to foot pedal and power).

Tuboplasty-Vasovasostomy

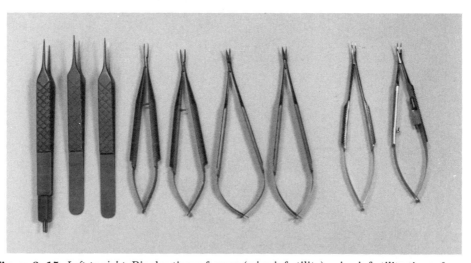

Figure 8–15. *Left to right.* Bipolar tissue forceps (microinfertility); microinfertility tissue forceps without teeth, microinfertility needle holder, curved and straight; microinfertility dissecting scissors, curved and straight; Castroviejo needle holder, and microinfertility needle holder with lock.

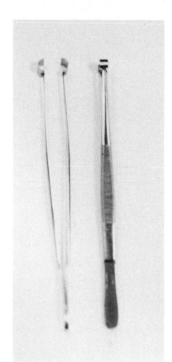

Figure 8–16. Microsurgery fallopian tube forceps.

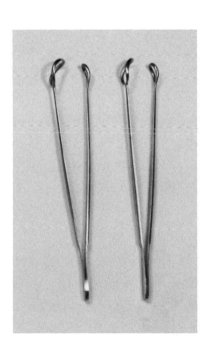

Figure 8–17. Ovary forceps.

CHAPTER 9

Ophthalmologic Surgery

Eye Specula

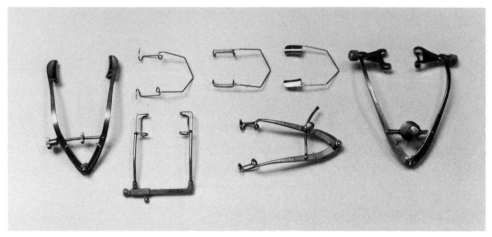

Figure 9–1. *Left to right.* Lancaster speculum, Murdock speculum, Knapp speculum, Maumenee-Park speculum without guard bar, *Top, left to right:* Barraquer-Kratz lid speculum. Barraquer child closed-blade speculum, and Barraquer solid-blade speculum.

Tissue Forceps

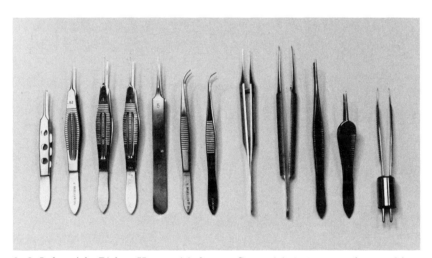

Figure 9–2. *Left to right.* Bishop-Harmon iris forceps, Castroviejo 0.12-mm teeth corneal forceps, 0.3-mm and 0.5-mm corneal forceps, jeweler's microforceps, two McPherson curved smooth-tip dressing forceps, straight Azar tying forceps, curved Kirby tying forceps, straight dressing forceps, Sauer or Paufique suture forceps, and McPherson microbipolar forceps.

Cataract Set

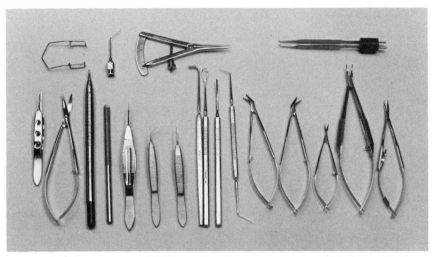

Figure 9–3. Cataract instrument set *(left to right):* Bishop-Harmon forceps, Wescott tenotomy scissors, ruby knife, beaver handle, 0.12-mm corneal forceps, angled and straight McPherson forceps, Javit muscle hook, Lewis lens scoop, iris spatula, Castroviejo cyclodialysis spatula, left corneal scissors, right corneal scissors, Vannas iridocapsulotomy scissors, Castroviejo angled locking needle holder, and Barraquer micro needleholder. *Top, left to right.* Barraquer wire lid speculum, irrigating 21-gauge needle cannula, Castroviejo caliper, and McPherson microbipolar forceps.

Accessories

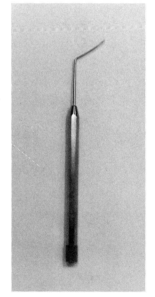

Figure 9–4. Castroviejo cyclodialysis sweep.

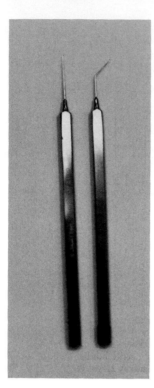

Figure 9–5. Sinskey lens positioner: straight and angled.

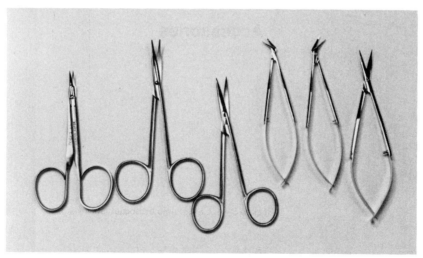

Figure 9–6. *Left to right.* Curved stitch scissors, Stevens tenotomy scissors, iris scissors, left corneal scissors, right corneal scissors, and Wescott tenotomy scissors.

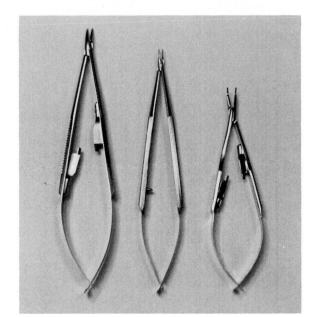

Figure 9–7. *Left to right.* Castroviejo micro needle holder, Torchia nonlocking needle holder, and McPherson locking needle holder.

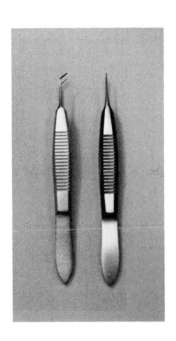

Figure 9–8. McPherson tying forceps: angled and straight.

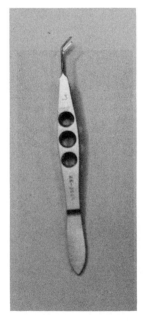

Figure 9–9. Bishop-Harmon 0.3 mm tissue forceps.

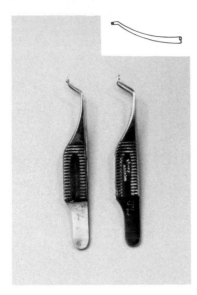

Figure 9–10. Corneal utility forceps (Colibri type). (*Inset* courtesy of Baxter Healthcare Corporation.)

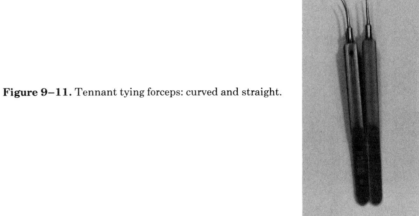

Figure 9–11. Tennant tying forceps: curved and straight.

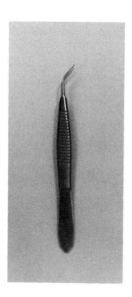

Figure 9–12. Long-angled McPherson capsule forceps.

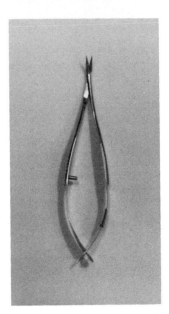

Figure 9–13. Vannas micro scissors.

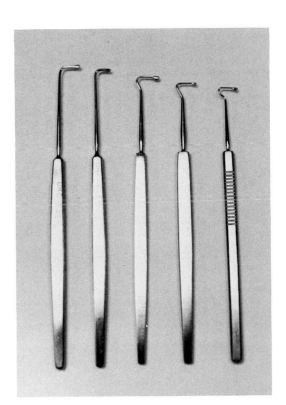

Figure 9–14. *Left to right.* Two Von Graefe strabismus hooks (large and medium) and three Jameson bulbous strabismus hooks.

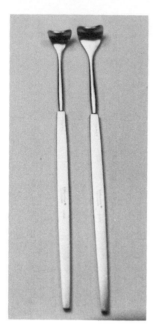

Figure 9–15. Desmarres lid retractors.

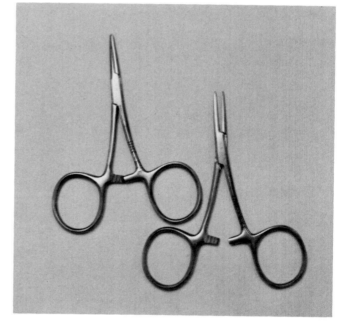

Figure 9–16. Hartman mosquito forceps.

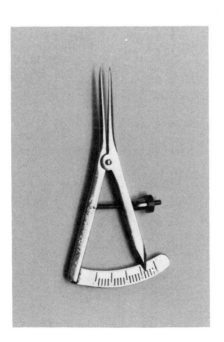

Figure 9–17. Castroviejo caliper.

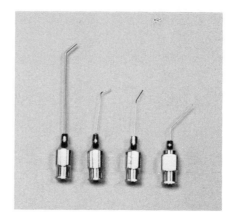

Figure 9–18. *Left to right.* Cyclodialysis irrigating cannula (21 gauge), air cannula (30 gauge), injection cannula (27 gauge), and long-angled irrigating cannula (25 gauge).

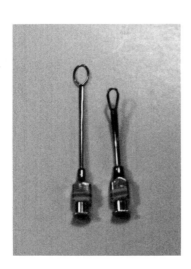

Figure 9–19. *Left.* Knolle-Pearce irrigating vectis. *Right.* Sheets irrigating vectis.

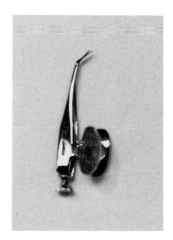

Figure 9–20. Barraquer-Dewecker iris scissors.

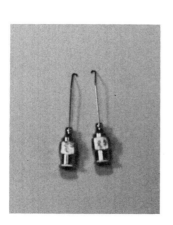

Figure 9–21. Hooked cannulas (22 gauge): left and right.

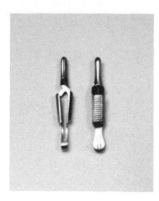

Figure 9–22. Serrefines.

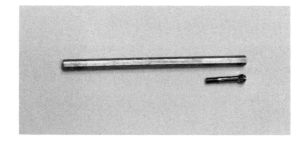

Figure 9–23. Chuck handle for Beaver blades (screw top).

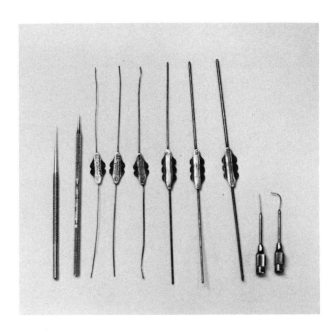

Figure 9–24. *Left to right.* Nettleship-Wilder lacrimal dilator, Muldoon lacrimal dilator, six lacrimal double-ended duct probes, straight and angled lacrimal irrigating cannulas (23 gauge).

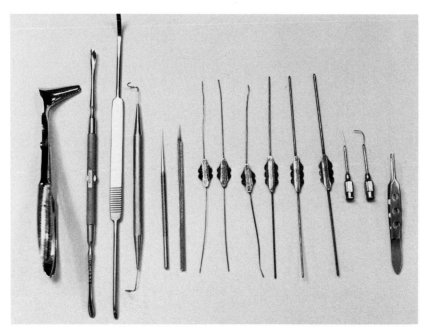

Figure 9–25. *Left to right.* Vienna nasal speculum, Freer elevator, Cottle elevator, pigtail probe, Nettleship-Wilder lacrimal dilator, Muldoon lacrimal dilator, six lacrimal double-ended duct probes, straight and angled lacrimal irrigating cannulas (23 gauge), and Bishop-Harmon forceps.

Keratoplasty

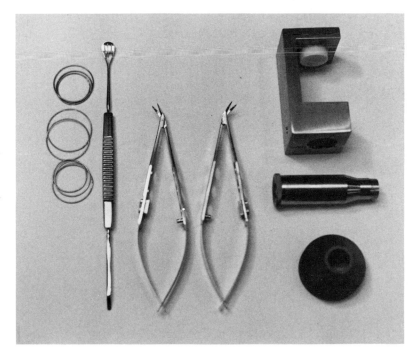

Figure 9–26. *Left to right.* Eight Flieringa fixation rings, Paton spatula and spoon, Troutman-Katzin corneal transplant scissors (left and right), Cottingham punch with universal handle, Teflon block, and Maloney keratometer.

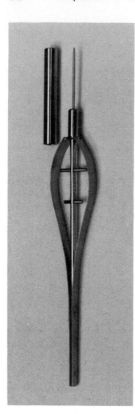

Figure 9–27. Haptic cutter.

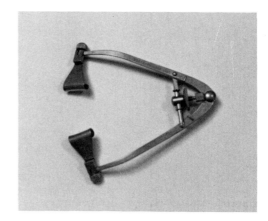

Figure 9–28. Lancaster lid speculum.

Blepharoplasty

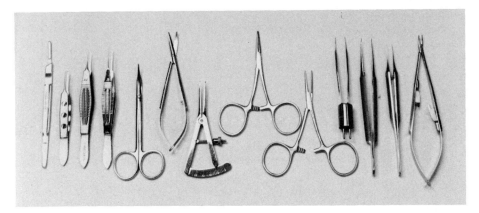

Figure 9–29. *Left to right.* No. 7 knife handle, Bishop-Harmon tissue forceps, Castroviejo tissue forceps (0.12-mm and 0.5 mm), Stevens tenotomy scissors, Wescott tenotomy scissors, Castroviejo caliper, Hartman mosquito clamps, McPherson microbipolar forceps, straight Azar tying forceps, Kirby curved tying forceps, and Castroviejo locking microneedle holder.

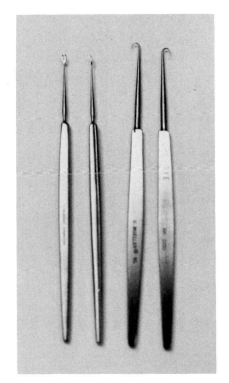

Figure 9–30. *Left.* Fixation hooks. *Right.* O'Connor sharp hooks.

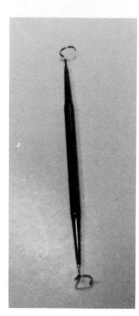

Figure 9–31. Pigtail probe.

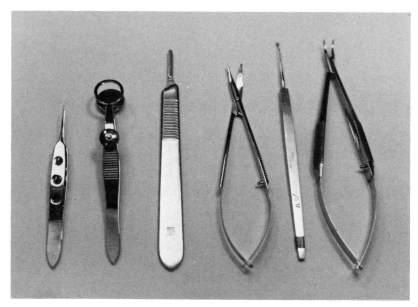

Figure 9–32. *Left to right.* Bishop-Harmon tissue forceps, Leahey chalazion clamp, No. 3 knife handle, Wescott tenotomy scissors, Meyhoeffer chalazion curette, and Barraquer microneedle holder.

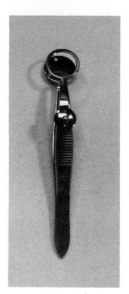

Figure 9–33. Leahey chalazion clamp.

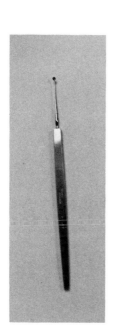

Figure 9–34. Meyhoeffer chalazion curette.

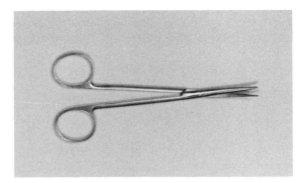

Figure 9–35. Stitch scissors.

Ear, Nose, and Throat Surgery

Minor Ear Surgery—Myringotomy

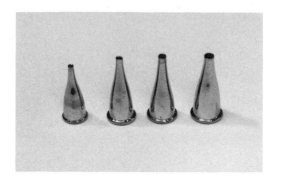

Figure 10–1. Gruber ear specula (assorted sizes).

Figure 10–2. Boucheron ear specula (assorted sizes).

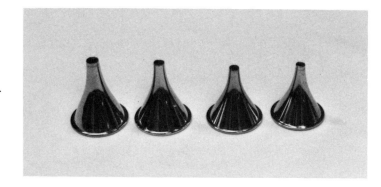

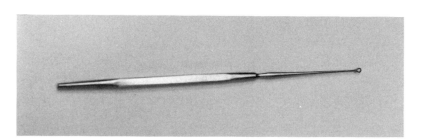

Figure 10–3. Freimuth ear curette (serrated loop).

Figure 10–4. Myringotomy knife spear blade and Universal handle.

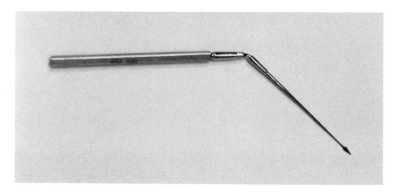

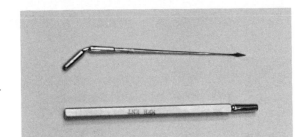

Figure 10–5. Myringotomy knife spear blade and Universal handle.

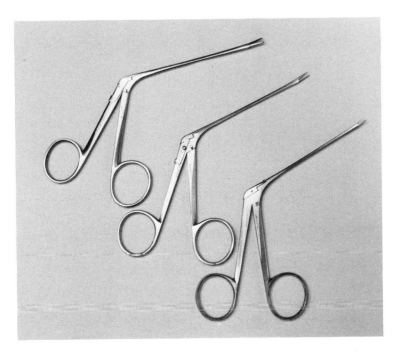

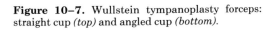

Figure 10–6. *Top to bottom.* Noyes ear forceps, House strut alligator forceps, and fine Wullstein forceps.

Figure 10–7. Wullstein tympanoplasty forceps: straight cup *(top)* and angled cup *(bottom)*.

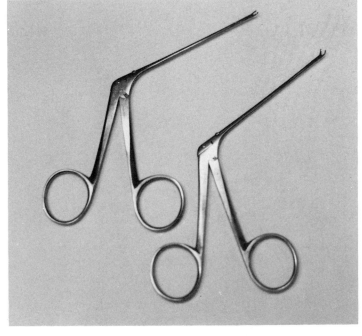

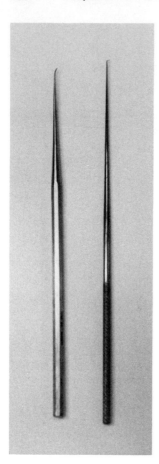

Figure 10–8. *Left.* Curved Rosen needle. *Right.* Day ear hook.

Figure 10–9. Two Brown cotton applicators and Lathbury cotton applicator.

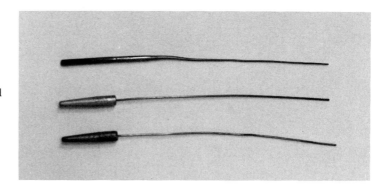

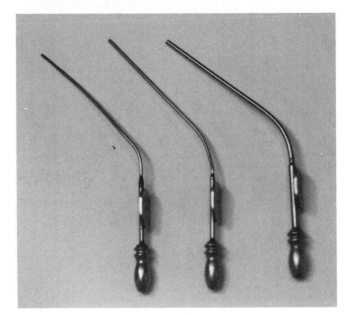

Figure 10–10. Baron suction tubes (Nos. 3, 5, and 7).

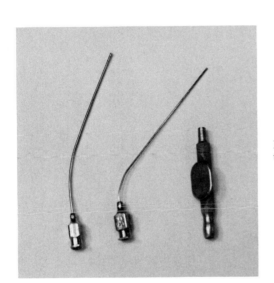

Figure 10–11. *Left.* Rosen suction tubes (Nos. 18 and 20). *Right.* House suction adapter.

Major Ear Surgery—Mastoidectomy

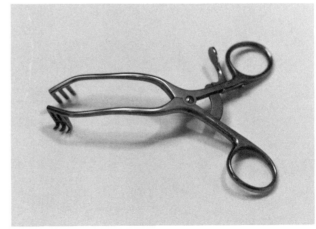

Figure 10–12. Schuknecht postauricular retractor.

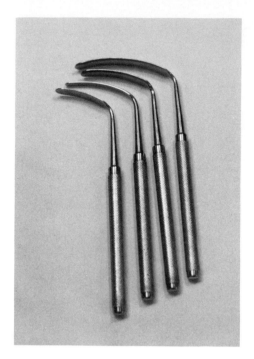

Figure 10–13. Sewall orbital retractors.

Figure 10–14. House suction tubes with irrigators (5 and 7 French).

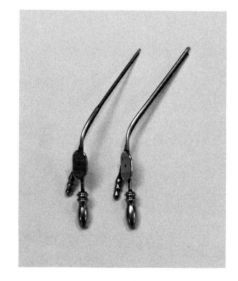

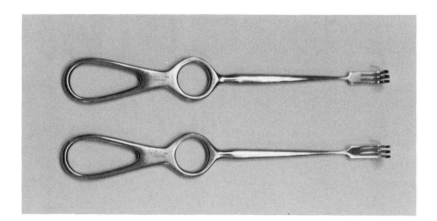

Figure 10–15. Lempert hand retractors.

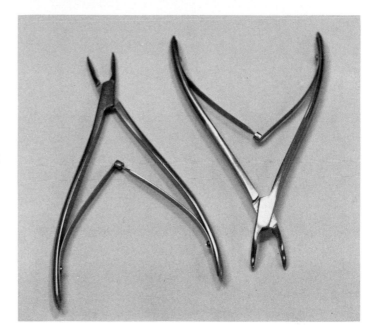

Figure 10–16. Lempert rongeurs: straight and angled.

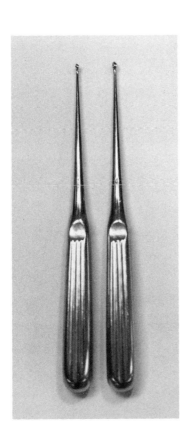

Figure 10–17. Lempert curettes, sizes 00 and 0.

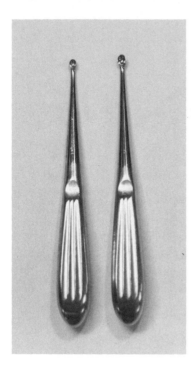

Figure 10–18. Spratt (Breen) mastoid curettes, sizes 1 and 2.

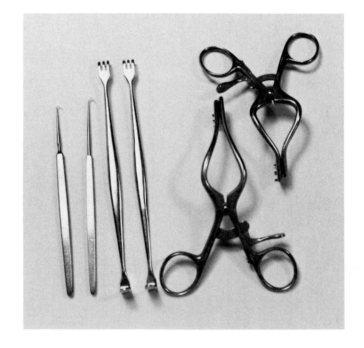

Figure 10–19. *Left to right.* Skin hook retractors, Senn retractors, and Wullstein retractors.

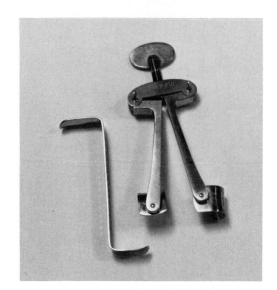

Figure 10–20. Henner retractor.

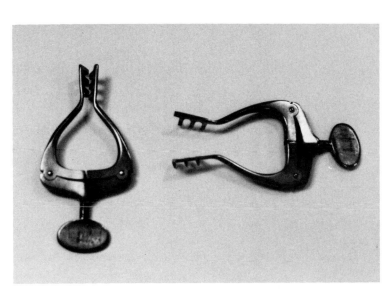

Figure 10–21. Jansen mastoid retractors.

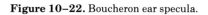

Figure 10–22. Boucheron ear specula.

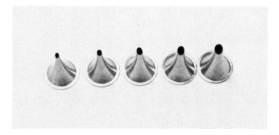

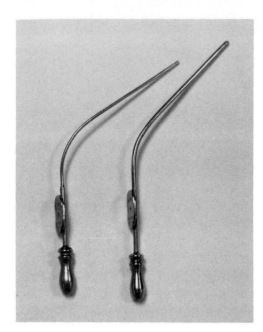

Figure 10–23. Baron suction tubes (Nos. 5 and 7).

Figure 10–24. Frazier suction tubes (Nos. 5 and 7).

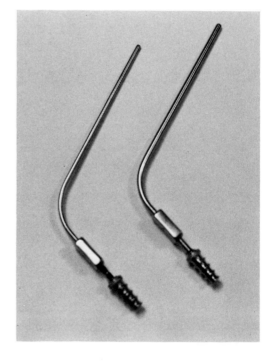

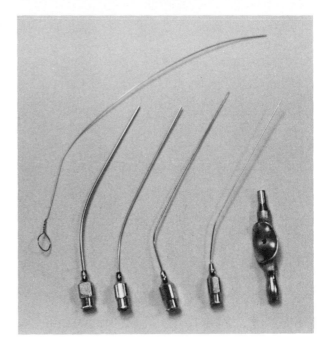

Figure 10–25. *Left to right.* Cleaning wire, Rosen suction tubes (Nos. 18, 20, 22, and 24), and House suction adapter.

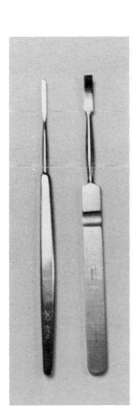

Figure 10–26. *Left.* Shambaugh elevator. *Right.* Lempert elevator.

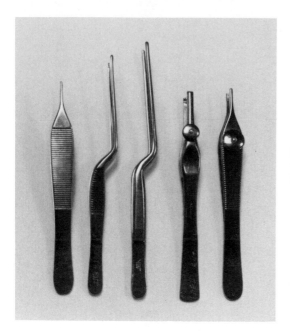

Figure 10–27. *Left to right.* Adson tissue forceps with teeth, Butler bayonet forceps, bayonet tissue forceps, Derlacki ossicle-holding clamp, and Sheehy ossicle-holding clamp.

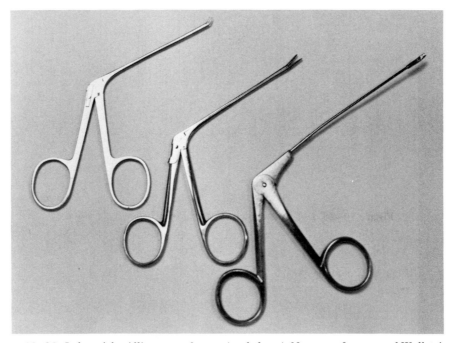

Figure 10–28. *Left to right.* Alligator ear forceps (angled cup), Noyes ear forceps, and Wullstein ear scissor.

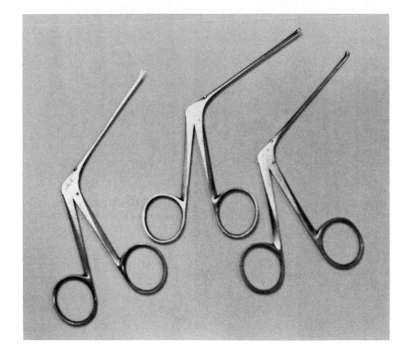

Figure 10–29. *Left to right.* Wullstein forceps (fine), Wullstein tympanic forceps (straight cup), and Wullstein tympanic forcep (angled cup).

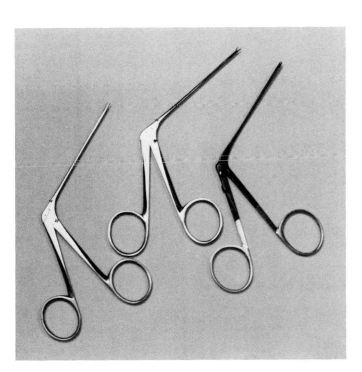

Figure 10–30. *Left to right.* Caparosa wire crimper, Schuknecht wire crimper, and middle ear scissors.

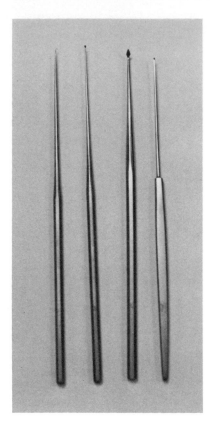

Figure 10–31. *Left to right.* Guilford-Wright stapes pick, Sheehy round knife, Hough incisional knife, and Shambaugh hook.

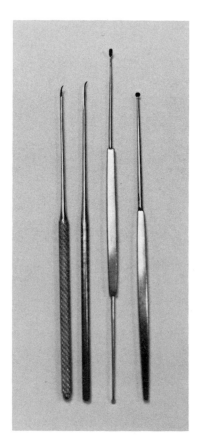

Figure 10–32. *Left to right.* Austin sickle knife, House myringotomy knife, McCabe flap knife dissector, and Rosen knife.

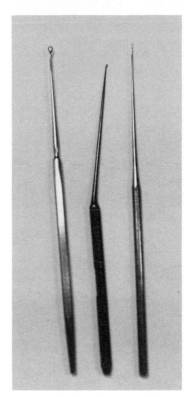

Figure 10–33. *Left to right.* Freimuth ear curette, Derlacki mobilizer, and House measuring rod.

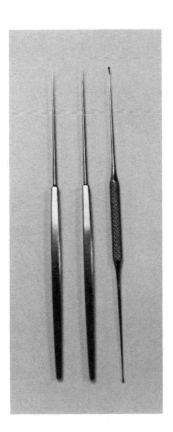

Figure 10–34. *Left to right.* House foot plate chisel, Shambaugh hook, and Tabb flap knife.

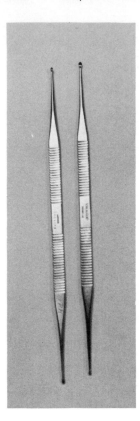

Figure 10–35. House stapes curettes.

Figure 10–36. *Left to right.* House middle ear mirror, House stapes curette, and McCabe perforation rasp.

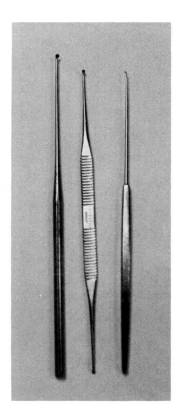

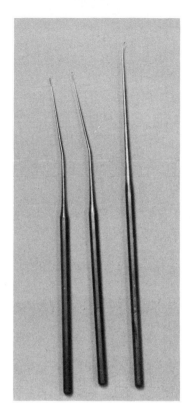

Figure 10–37. *Left to right.* Hough pick, Hough evacuator, and House-Rosen needle.

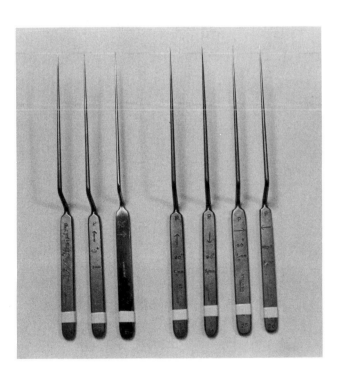

Figure 10–38. Kos picks.

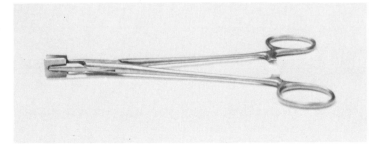

Figure 10–39. House Gelfoam pressure forceps.

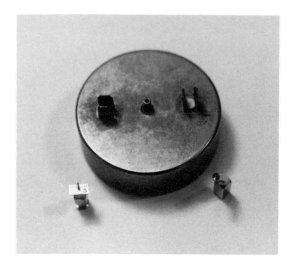

Figure 10–40. Wire bending die.

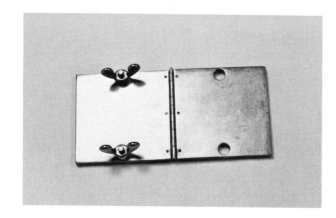

Figure 10–41. Paparella tissue press.

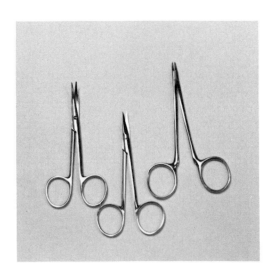

Figure 10–42. *Left to right.* Stevens tenotomy scissors, Joseph scissors, and malleus nipper.

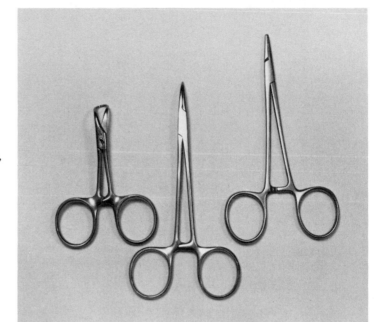

Figure 10–43. *Left to right.* Backhaus towel forceps, mosquito hemostat, and Webster needle holder.

Nasal Surgery

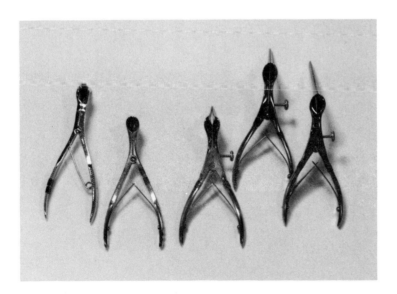

Figure 10–44. *Left to right.* Storz-Vienna nasal speculum, Vienna nasal speculum, and three Cottle nasal specula.

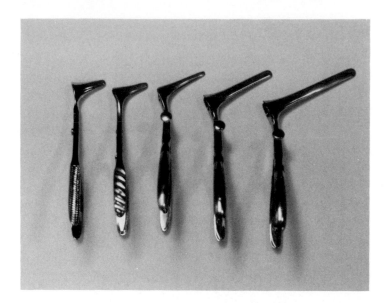

Figure 10–45. *Left to right.* Storz-Vienna nasal speculum, Vienna nasal speculum, three Cottle nasal specula.

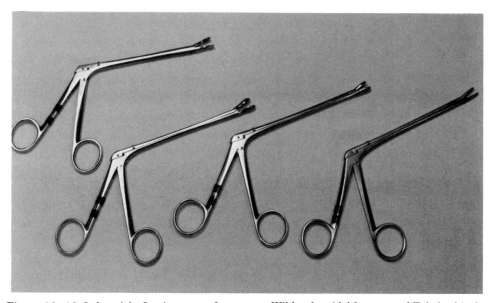

Figure 10–46. *Left to right.* Lewis septum forceps, two Wilde ethmoidal forceps, and Takahashi ethmoidal forceps.

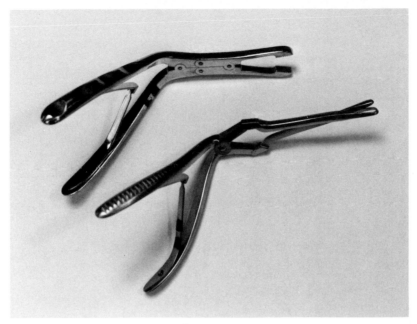

Figure 10–47. *Top.* Septum morselizer forceps. *Bottom.* Jansen-Middleton septum forceps.

Figure 10–48. *Left to right.* Curved Mayo scissors, wire scissors, Metzenbaum scissors, Foman lateral scissors, and straight Mayo scissors.

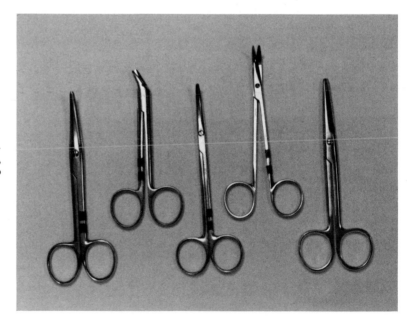

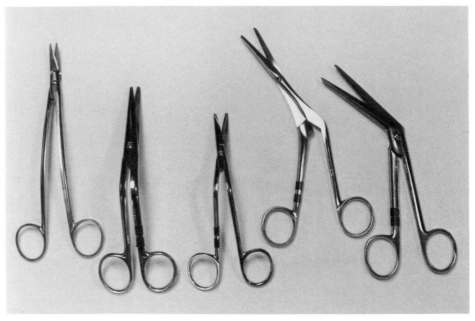

Figure 10–49. *Left to right.* Goldman upper lateral scissors, Foman dorsal scissors, Lakeside model nasal scissors, Knight nasal scissors, and Seiler turbinate scissors.

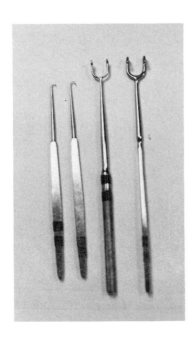

Figure 10–50. *Left to right.* Two skin hooks, Cottle sharp double hook and Foman retractor.

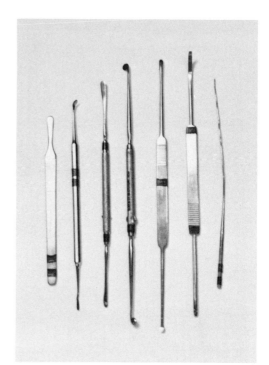

Figure 10–51. *Left to right.* Cottle nasal knife, Woodson elevator, Freer double-ended elevator, Pierce submucosa dissector, Cottle double-ended septum elevator, Cottle elevator, and Lathbury applicator.

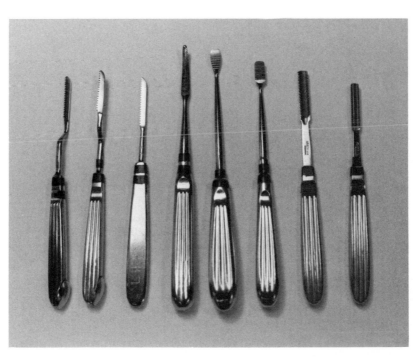

Figure 10–52. *Left to right.* Two Joseph angled nasal saws, Joseph straight nasal saw, Stratte naso-frontal rasp, Lewis rasp, Israel rasp, and Maltz rasp.

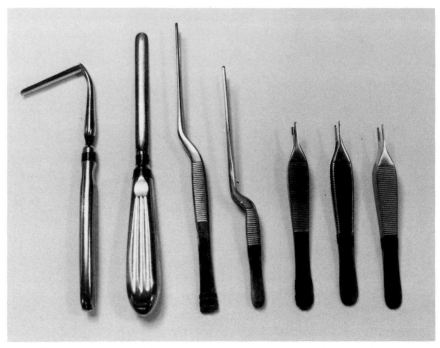

Figure 10–53. *Left to right.* Aufricht nasal retractor, Boies nasal fracture elevator, bayonet tissue forceps (long and short), Brown-Adson tissue forceps, Adson tissue forceps with teeth, and Adson tissue forceps without teeth.

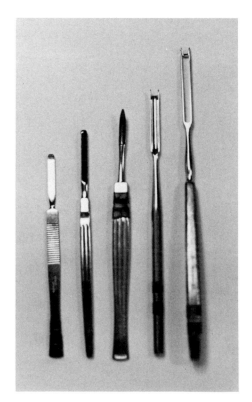

Figure 10–54. *Left to right.* McKenty periosteal elevator, Joseph button-end knife, Cottle double-edge knife, Ballenger chisel, and Ballenger swivel knife.

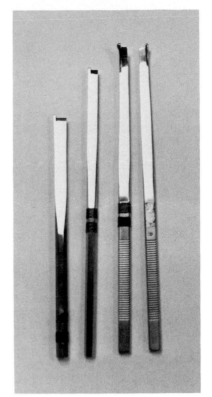

Figure 10–55. *Left.* Foman guarded osteotomes. *Right.* Anderson-Neivert osteotomes.

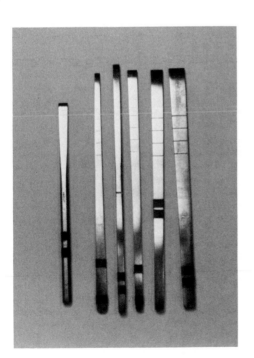

Figure 10–56. *Left.* Sheehan osteotome. *Right.* Five Cottle osteotomes.

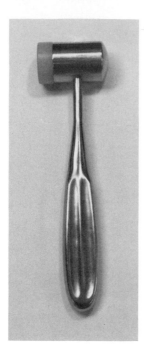

Figure 10–57. Cottle mallet.

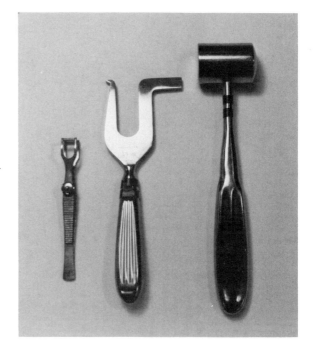

Figure 10–58. *Left to right.* Cottle columella clamp, Rubin naso-frontal osteotome, and lead-filled mallet.

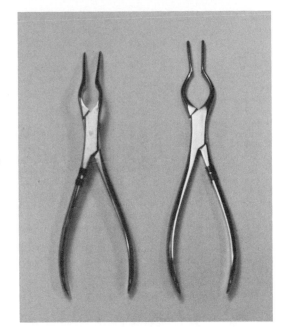

Figure 10–59. *Left.* Asch septum-straightening forceps. *Right.* Walsham septum-straightening forceps.

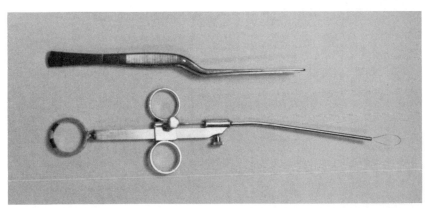

Figure 10–60. *Left.* Bayonet dressing forceps. *Right.* Krause nasal snare (with nasal snare wire).

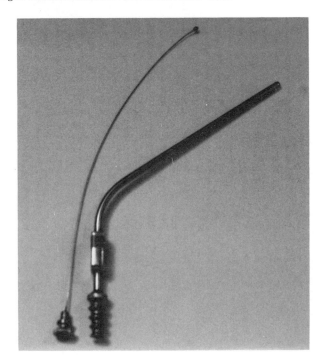

Figure 10–61. Frazier suction tube with stylet.

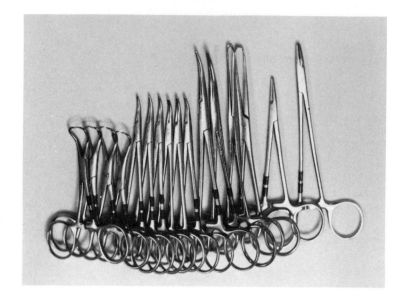

Figure 10–62. *Left to right.* Four Backhaus towel clamps, six curved mosquito clamps, two Kelly forceps, two Allis forceps, Webster needle holder, and Mayo-Hegar needle holder.

Tonsillectomy and Adenoidectomy

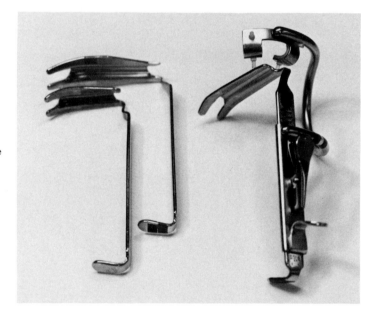

Figure 10–63. Davis-Crowe mouth gag with three interchangeable tongue depressors.

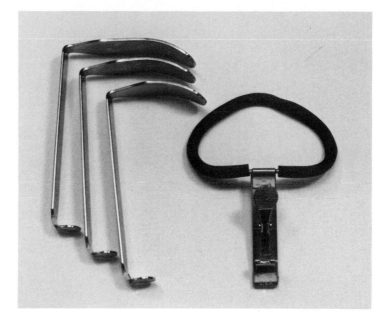

Figure 10–64. McIvor mouth gag with three tongue blades.

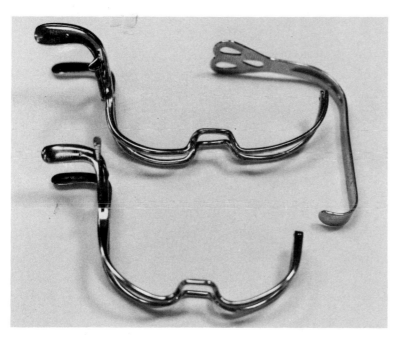

Figure 10–65. Jennings mouth gags (large and medium) and Wieder tongue depressor.

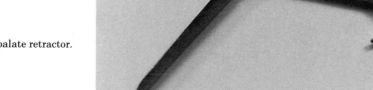

Figure 10–66. Jackson palate retractor.

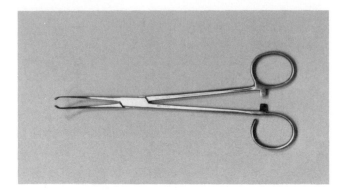

Figure 10–67. White tonsil grasping forceps.

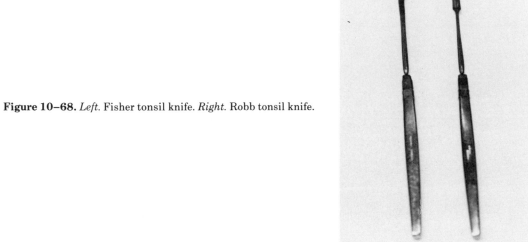

Figure 10–68. *Left.* Fisher tonsil knife. *Right.* Robb tonsil knife.

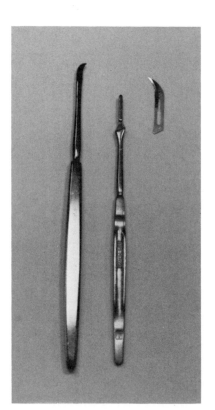

Figure 10–69. *Left.* Canfield tonsil knife. *Right.* No. 7 handle with No. 12 blade.

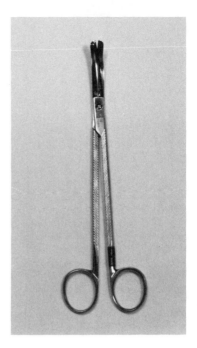

Figure 10–70. Good tonsil scissors.

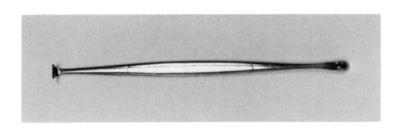

Figure 10–71. Hurd tonsil dissector (pillar retractor).

Figure 10–72. Laryngeal mirror.

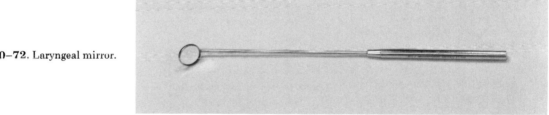
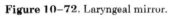

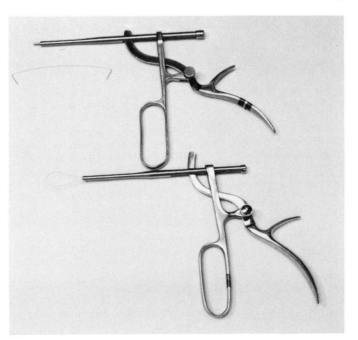

Figure 10–73. Tydings snares with No. 8 wire.

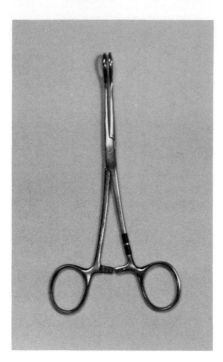

Figure 10–74. Ballenger sponge forceps.

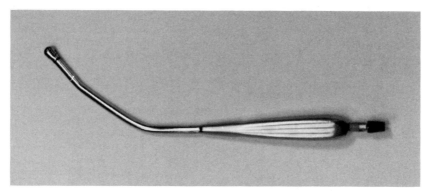

Figure 10–75. Yankauer suction tube.

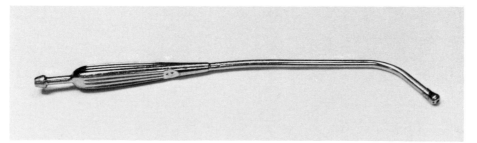

Figure 10–76. Pynchon suction tube.

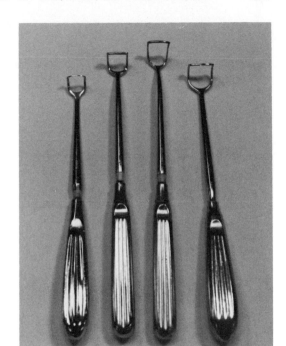

Figure 10–77. Barnhill adenoid curettes.

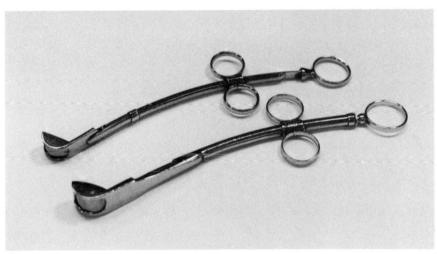

Figure 10–78. LaForce adenotomes.

Tracheotomy

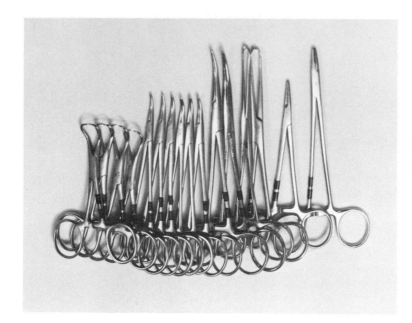

Figure 10–79. *Left to right.* Four towel clips, six mosquito clamps, two curved Kelly clamps, two Allis clamps, Webster needle holder, and Mayo needle holder.

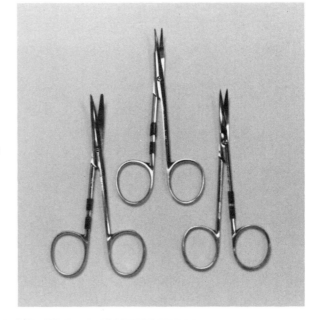

Figure 10–80. *Left to right.* Small Metzenbaum scissors, Stevens tenotomy scissors, and iris scissors.

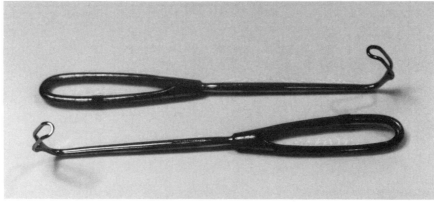

Figure 10–81. Cushing retractors.

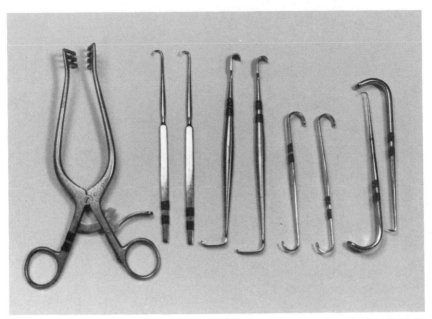

Figure 10–82. *Left to right.* Weitlaner retractor, Graham-Blount tracheal hooks, Senn-Dingman retractors, Luer S-shaped tracheal retractors, and Jackson tracheal tenacula.

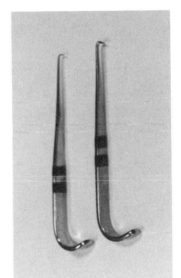

Figure 10–83. Jackson tracheal tenacula.

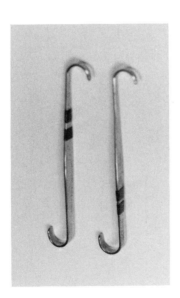

Figure 10–84. Luer S-shaped tracheal retractors.

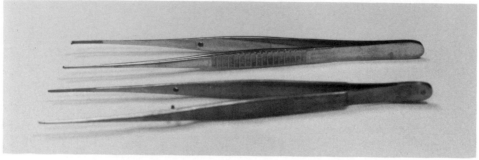

Figure 10–85. Potts-Smith tissue forceps, with and without teeth.

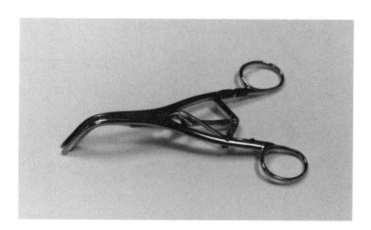

Figure 10–86. LaBorde tracheal dilator.

Figure 10–87. *Left.* Trousseau-Jackson dilator. *Right.* LaBorde tracheal dilator.

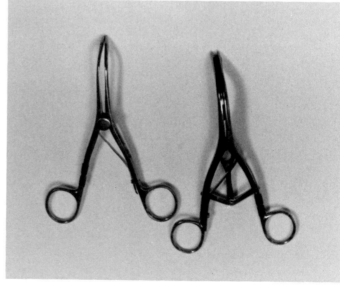

Thyroidectomy

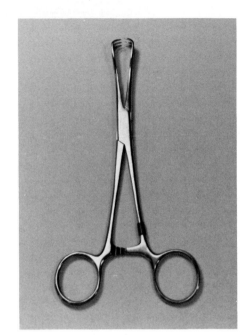

Figure 10–88. Lahey clamp.

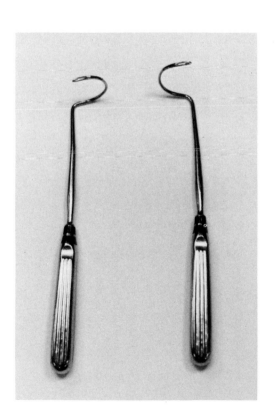

Figure 10–89. Deschamps ligature carriers.

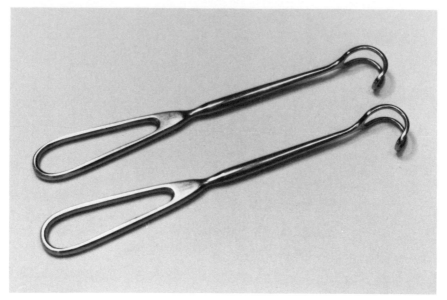

Figure 10–90. Green retractors.

Endoscopic Surgery

Arthroscopy

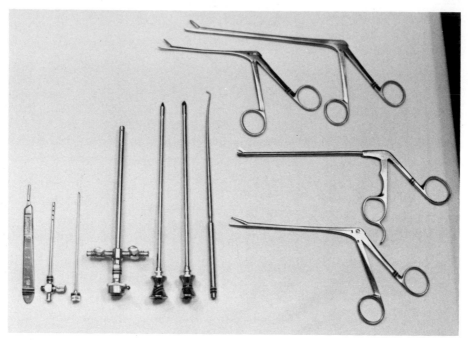

Figure 11–1. *Left to right.* No. 3 knife handle, egress cannula with angled trocar, arthroscope sheath, blunt and sharp trocar, and Dandy nerve hook (probe). *Top to bottom.* Takahashi forceps (long and short), hook scissors, and Hoen forceps (rat-tooth).

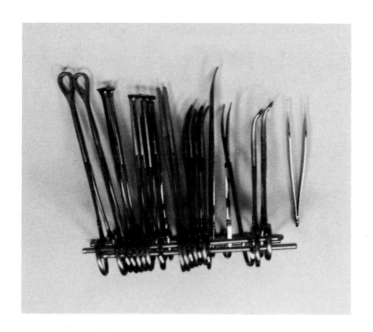

Figure 11–2. *Left to right.* Two sponge forceps, two Adair-Allis forceps, four Allis clamps, two Kocher clamps, four Crile clamps, regular and short Metzenbaum scissors, two towel clips, and Adson forceps with teeth.

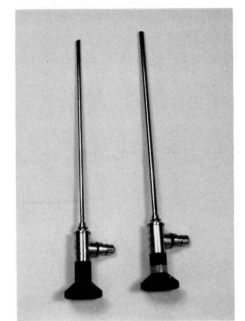

Figure 11–3. *Left.* 25° telescope. *Right.* 30° telescope.

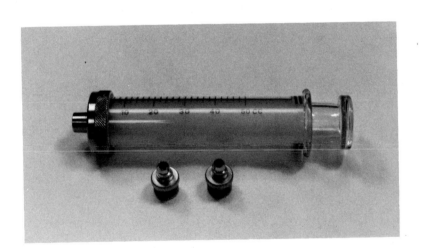

Figure 11–4. Toomey syringe with adapters.

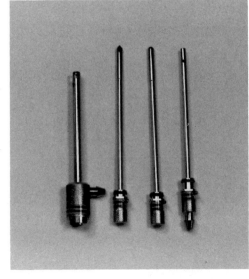

Figure 11–5. Zimmer irrigation cannulas with sharp and blunt trocars.

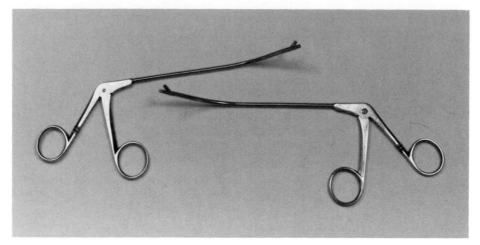

Figure 11–6. Basket forceps: right curved and left curved.

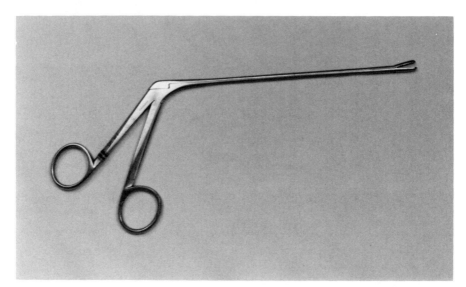

Figure 11–7. Takahashi forceps.

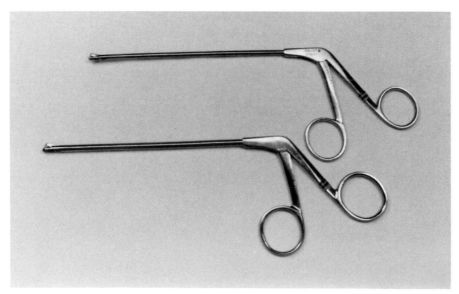

Figure 11–8. Hook scissors, 3.4 mm and 4.5 mm straight.

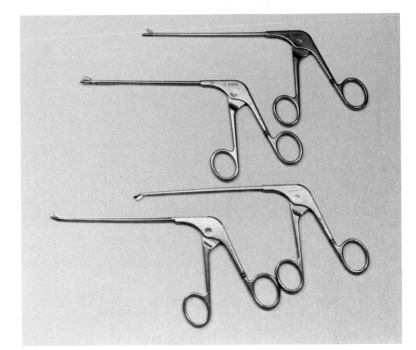

Figure 11–9. Acufex punch forceps *(top to bottom):* 2.7 mm, 3.4 mm, 1.3 mm (down-biter), and 1.5 mm.

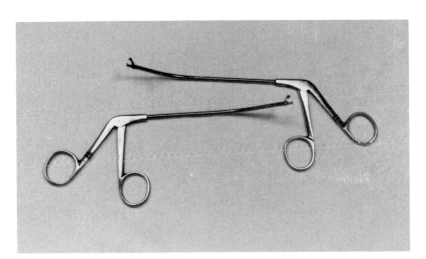

Figure 11–10. Hook scissors: right curved and left curved.

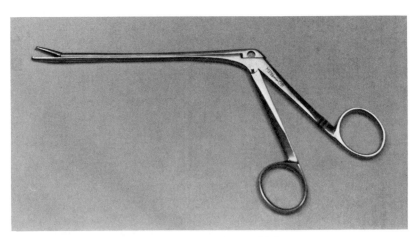

Figure 11–11. Hoen (rat-tooth) forceps.

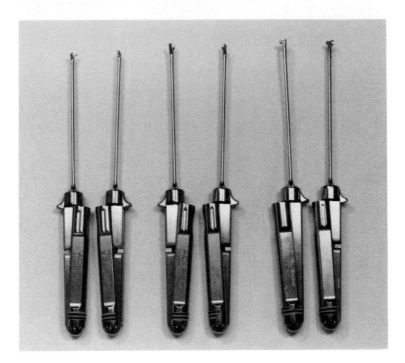

Figure 11–12. *Left to right.* Acufex rotary hook scissors: 60° right and left and 20° right and left; Acufex rotary basket punch 90° right and left.

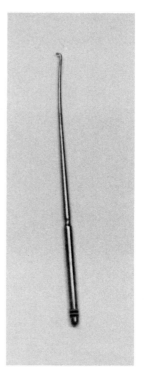
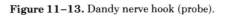

Figure 11–13. Dandy nerve hook (probe).

Cystoscopy

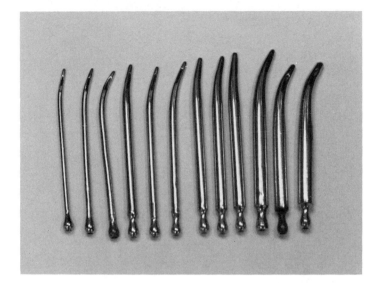

Figure 11–14. Walther female dilators.

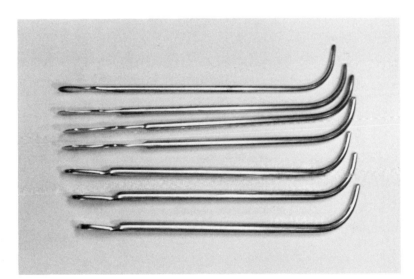

Figure 11–15. Van Buren urethral sounds (dilators).

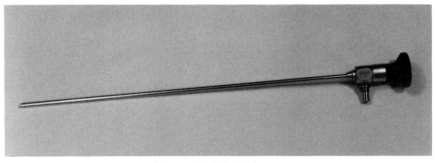

Figure 11–16. 0° telescope.

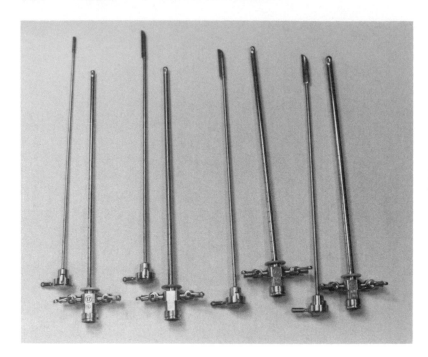

Figure 11-17. Cystoscope sheaths with obturators: sizes 17, 20, 22, and 25.

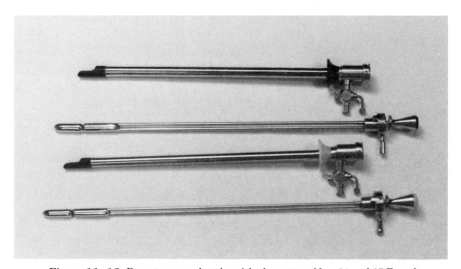

Figure 11-18. Resectoscope sheaths with obturators: Nos. 24 and 27 French.

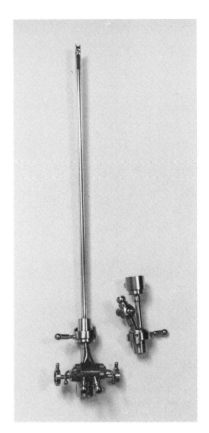

Figure 11-19. Catheter deflecting mechanism with telescope bridge.

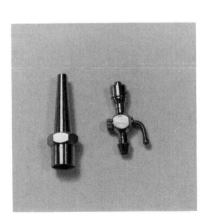

Figure 11-20. *Left.* Cone-Toomey syringe adapter. *Right.* Luer-Lok stopcock water adapter.

Figure 11-21. *Left to right.* Cystoscopy rubber tips, Luer-Lok adapter, and ureteral catheter adapter.

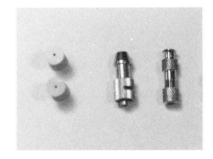

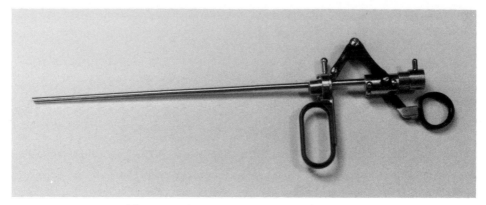

Figure 11–22. Resectoscope working element.

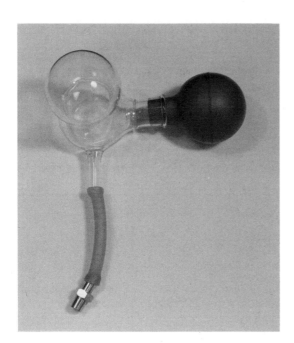

Figure 11–23. Ellik evacuator.

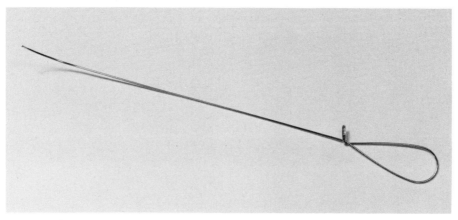

Figure 11–24. Mandrin (catheter guide).

Hysteroscopy

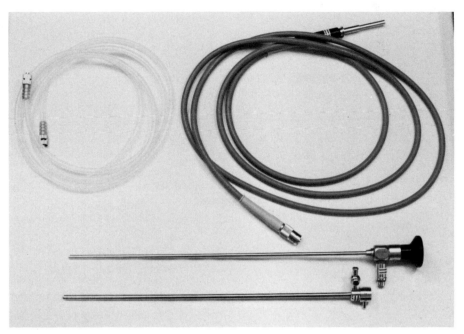

Figure 11–25. Silastic tubing, light source cord, 30° telescope, and insufflation channel with stopcock.

Laparoscopy

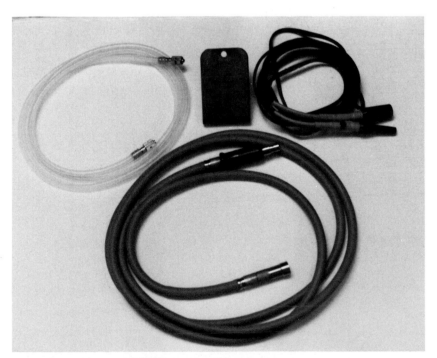

Figure 11–26. *Left to right.* Top: Silastic insufflation tubing two Luer-Lok connectors, cord clip, bipolar cautery cord, and light source cord.

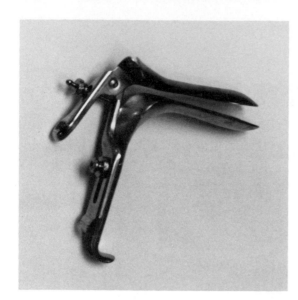

Figure 11–27. Graves vaginal speculum.

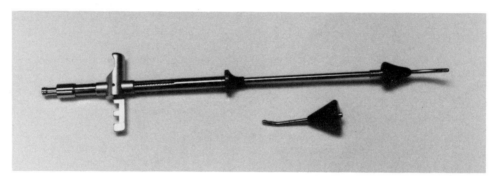

Figure 11–28. Cohen-Eder cannula with large and small acorns and insufflation channel.

Figure 11–29. Verres needles: 10 cm, 12 cm, and 15 cm.

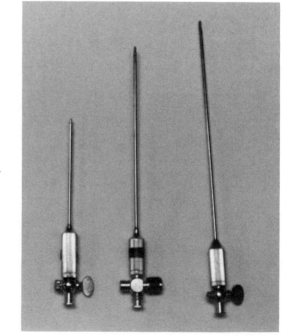

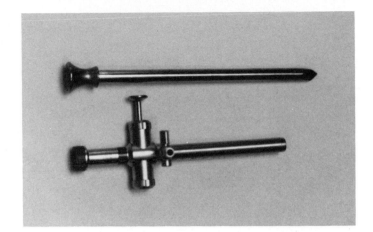

Figure 11–30. Piston valve cannula (10 mm) with sealing cap and trocar.

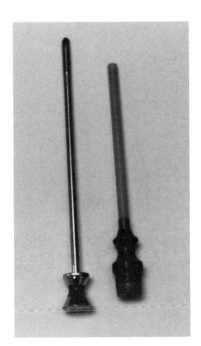

Figure 11–31. Trocar (5 mm) with cannula.

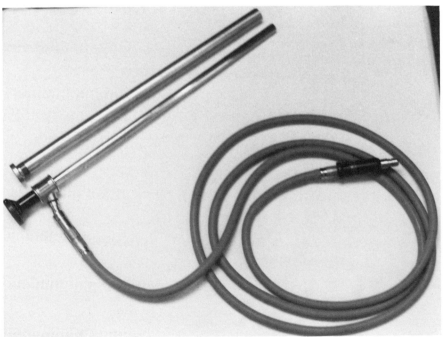

Figure 11–32. 0° telescope with light cord and warming cannula.

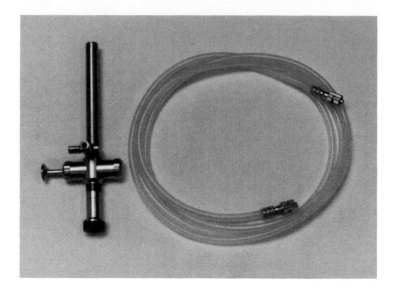

Figure 11-33. Trocar (10 mm) with insufflation tubing.

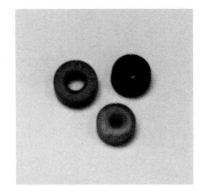

Figure 11-34. Sealing caps.

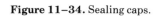

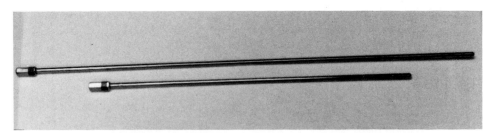

Figure 11-35. Probes: 18 inches and 12.5 inches.

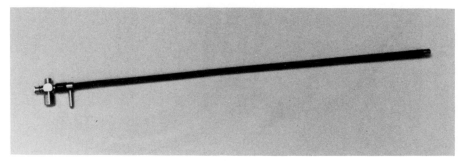

Figure 11-36. Cautery tip.

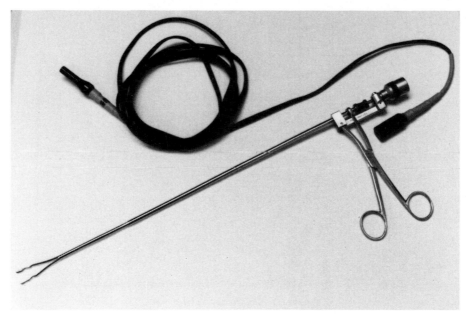

Figure 11–37. Kleppinger forceps with cord.

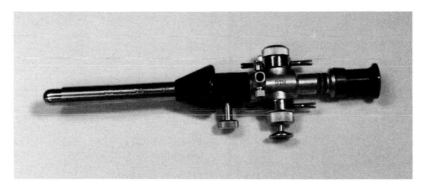

Figure 11–38. Hasson laparoscopy cannula with obturator and cone sleeve.

Figure 11–39. Hasson laparoscopy cannula with obturator and cone sleeve.

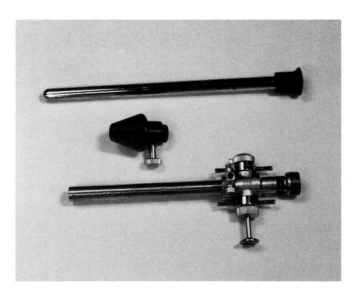

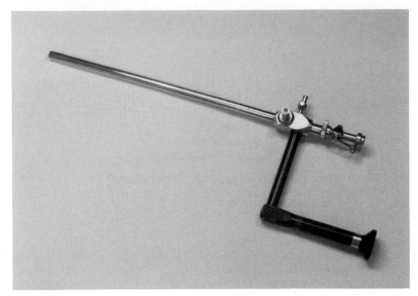

Figure 11–40. Operating telescope.

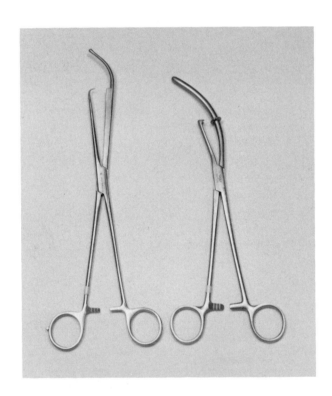

Figure 11–41. *Left.* Hulka tenaculum. *Right.* Sargis tenaculum.

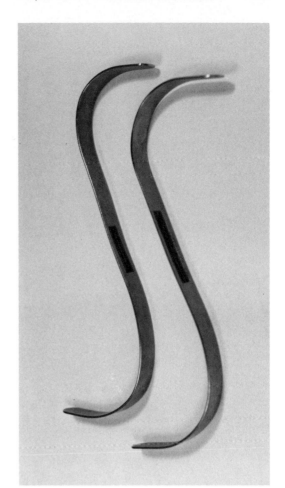

Figure 11–42. S-shaped retractors.

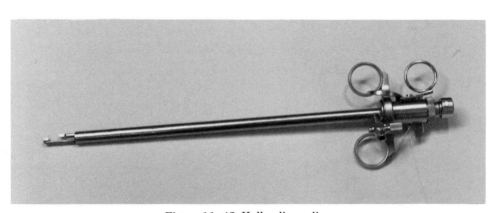

Figure 11–43. Hulka clip applier.

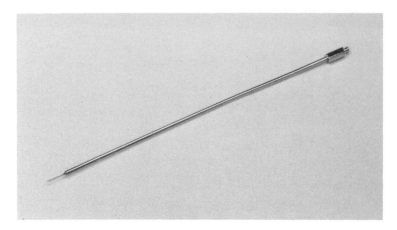

Figure 11–44. Hasson ovarian needle.

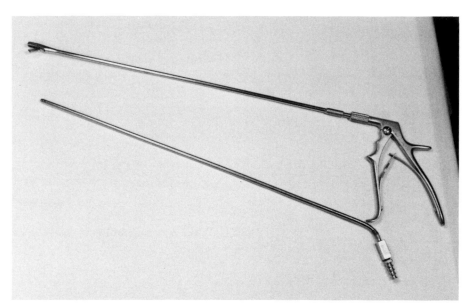

Figure 11–45. Laparoscopy biopsy forceps with suction tube.

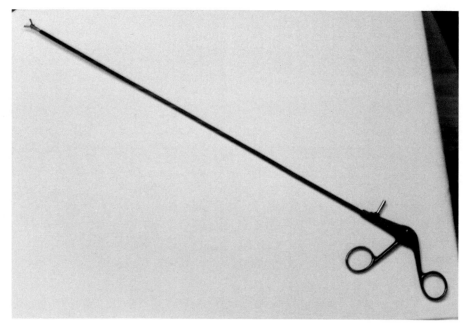

Figure 11–46. Laparoscopy biopsy forceps.

Bronchoscopy

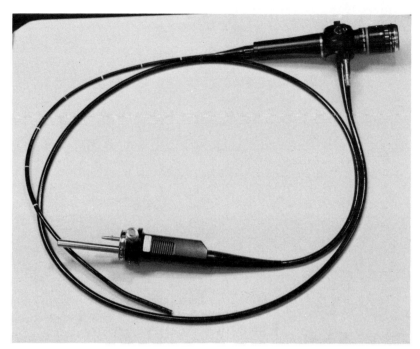

Figure 11–47. Flexible bronchoscope.

Laryngoscopy

Figure 11–48. Jackson laryngoscope with fiberoptic light carrier.

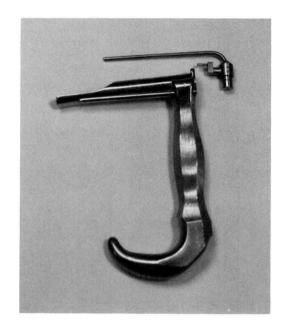

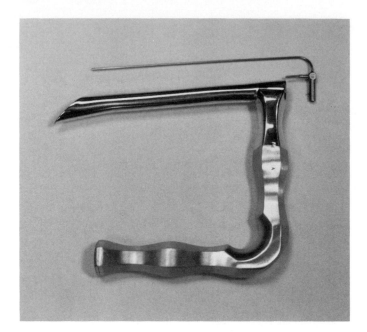

Figure 11–49. Holinger laryngoscope with fiberoptic light carrier.

Esophagoscopy

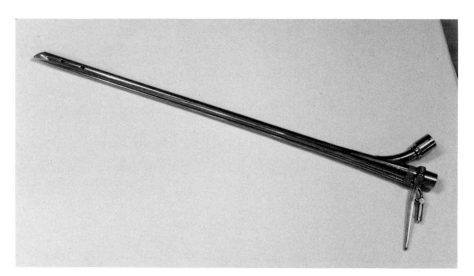

Figure 11–50. Holinger esophagoscope with fiberoptic light carrier.

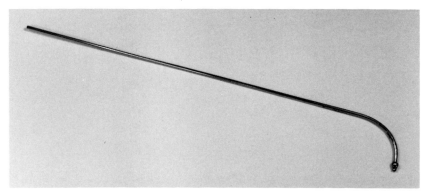

Figure 11–51. Jackson open-end aspirating tube.

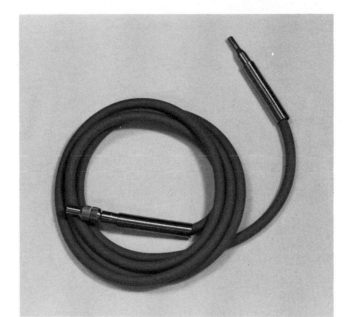

Figure 11–52. Fiberoptic light cord.

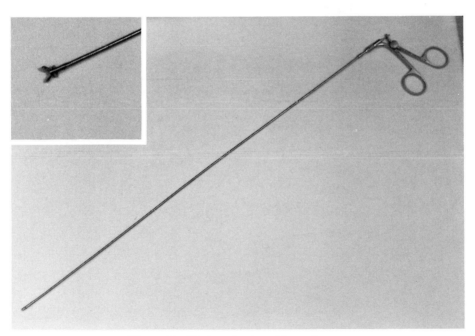

Figure 11–53. Broncheal cup biopsy forceps.

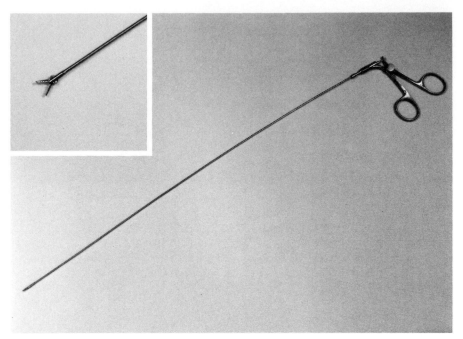

Figure 11–54. Kahler broncheal grasping forceps.

Sigmoidoscopy

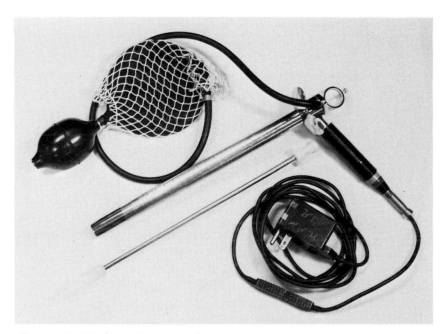

Figure 11–55. Sigmoidoscopy with obturator and electrical adapter.

Pediatric Surgery

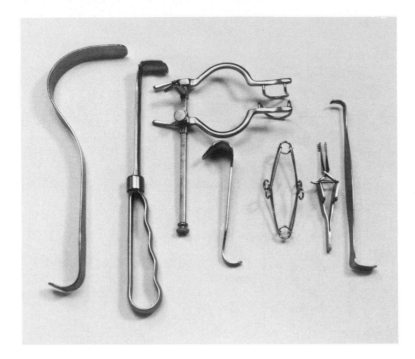

Figure 12–1. *Left to right.* Baby Deaver retractor, small Richardson retractor, pediatric Balfour retractor with blade, baby spring wire retractors, Heiss retractor, and Childrens' Hospital retractor.

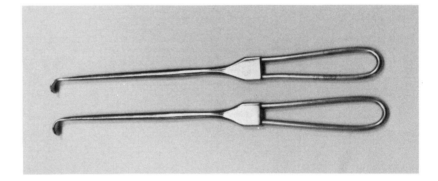

Figure 12–2. Vein retractors.

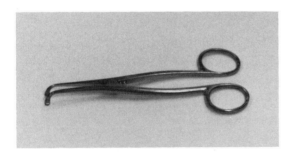

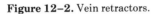

Figure 12–3. Ravich stenosis spreader.

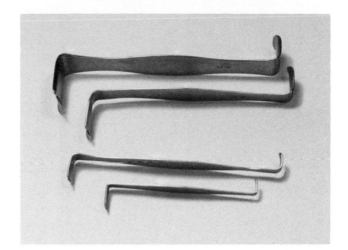

Figure 12–4. *Top.* Crile retractors. *Bottom.* Childrens' Hospital retractors.

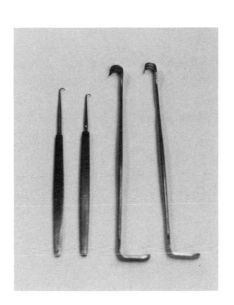

Figure 12–5. Skin hooks and Senn retractors.

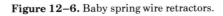

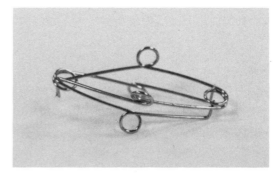

Figure 12–6. Baby spring wire retractors.

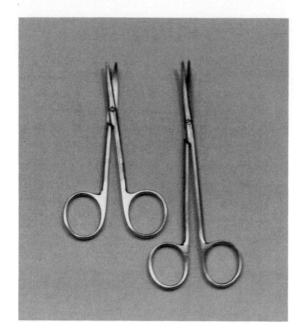

Figure 12–7. *Left.* Curved strabismus scissors. *Right.* Small Metzenbaum scissors.

Figure 12–8. Webster needle holder.

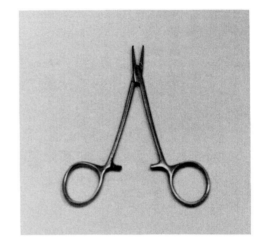

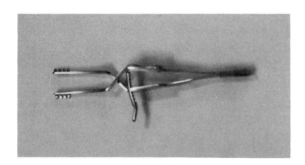

Figure 12–9. Heiss retractor.

CHAPTER

13

Orthopedic Surgery

Minor Orthopedic Surgery

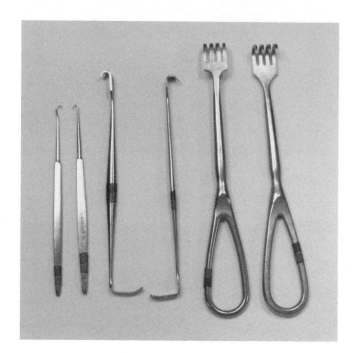

Figure 13–1. *Left to right.* Skin hooks, Senn retractors, and rake (Volkmann) retractors.

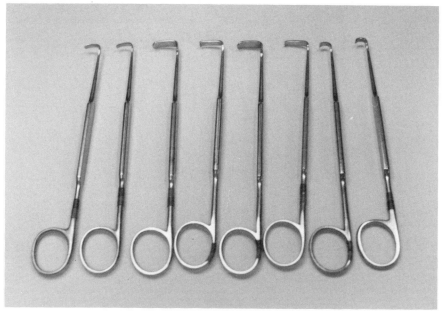

Figure 13–2. Meyerding finger retractors with assorted blades.

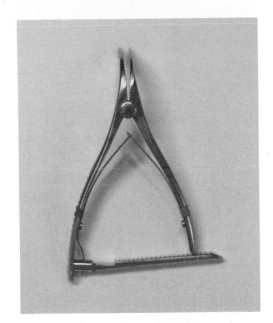

Figure 13–3. Inge lamina spreader.

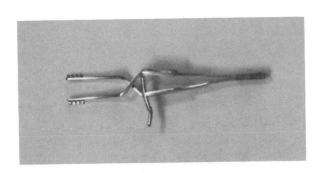

Figure 13–4. Heiss retractor.

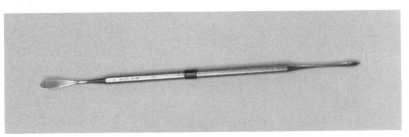

Figure 13–5. Freer elevator.

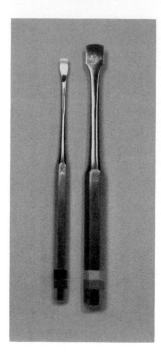

Figure 13–6. Key periosteal elevators.

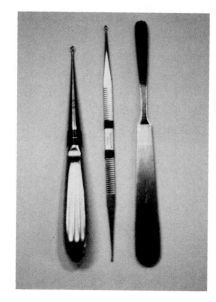

Figure 13–7. *Left to right.* Brun (Spratt) curette size 3-0; House curette (double-ended) and Maltz-Lipsett nasal rasp.

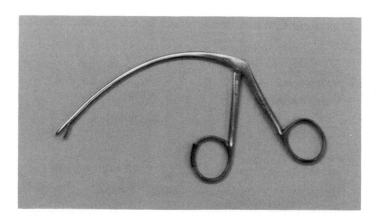

Figure 13–8. Carroll tendon-passing forceps.

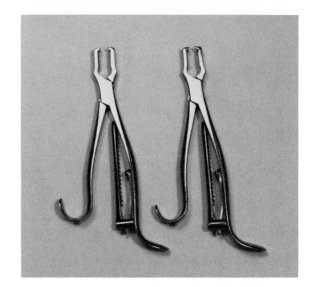

Figure 13–9. Kern bone-holding forceps.

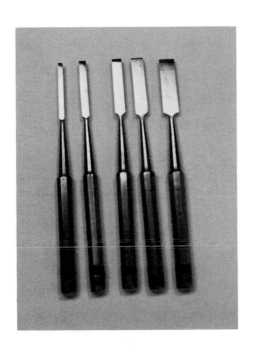

Figure 13–10. Hoke osteotomes.

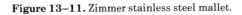

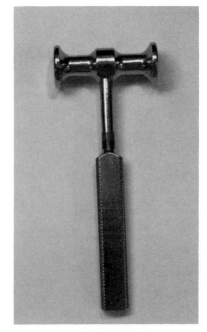

Figure 13–11. Zimmer stainless steel mallet.

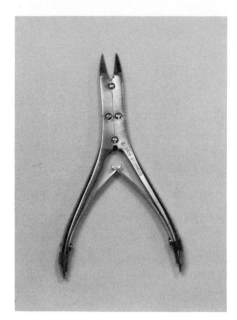

Figure 13–12. Zimmer bone cutting forceps (double action).

Figure 13–13. Kleinert-Kutz bone rongeur (double action).

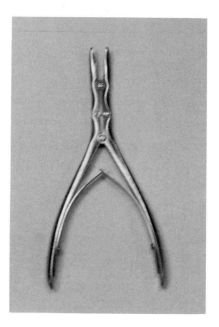

Shoulder Surgery

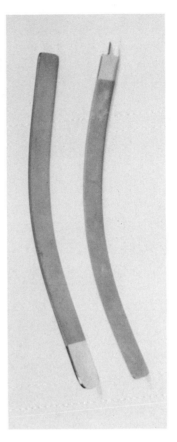

Figure 13–14. *Left.* Bankart muscle retractor. *Right.* Rowe capsule retractor.

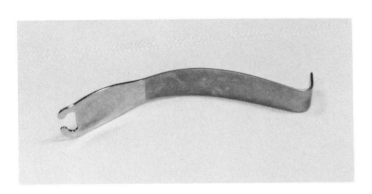

Figure 13–15. Bankart humeral head retractor.

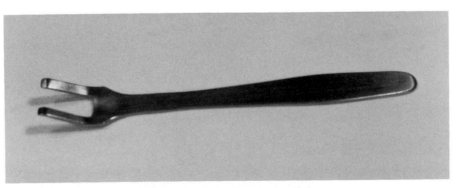

Figure 13–16. Bankart capsule fork.

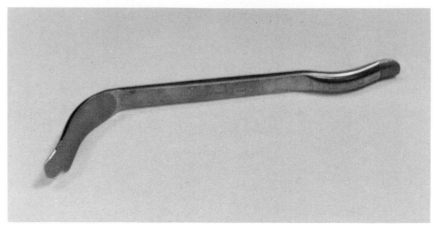

Figure 13–17. Bankart bone skid.

Knee Surgery

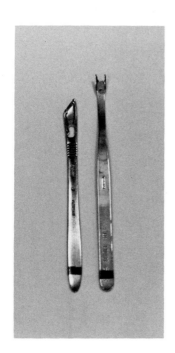

Figure 13–18. *Left.* Beaver knife handle. *Right.* Stryker cartilage knife.

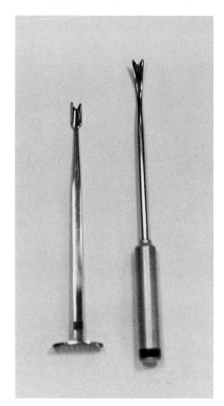

Figure 13–19. *Left.* Smillie cartilage knife. *Right.* Downing cartilage knife.

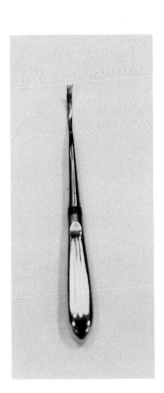

Figure 13–20. Smith posterior cartilage stripper.

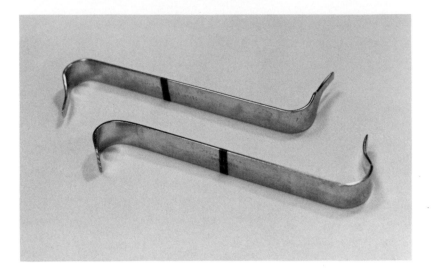

Figure 13–21. Blount knee retractors.

Figure 13–22. Myers knee retractor.

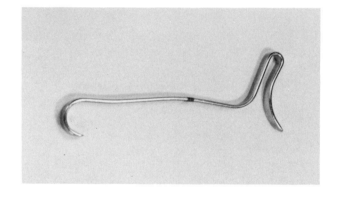

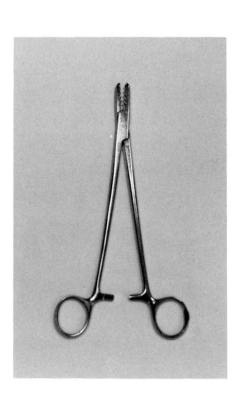

Figure 13–23. Martin cartilage clamp.

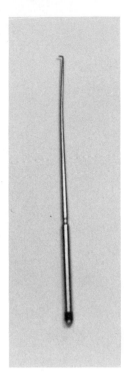

Figure 13–24. Dandy nerve hook.

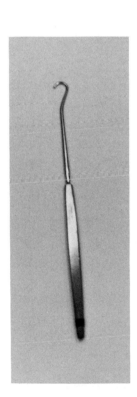

Figure 13–25. Graham nerve hook.

Major Orthopedic Surgery

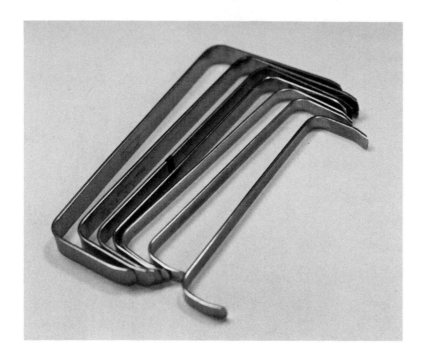

Figure 13–26. Sofield retractors.

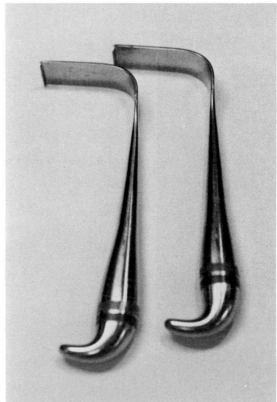

Figure 13–27. Meyerding retractors.

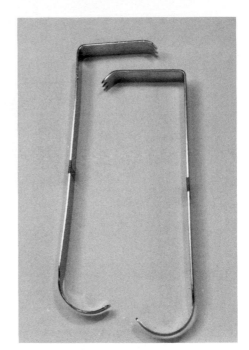

Figure 13–28. Hibbs retractors.

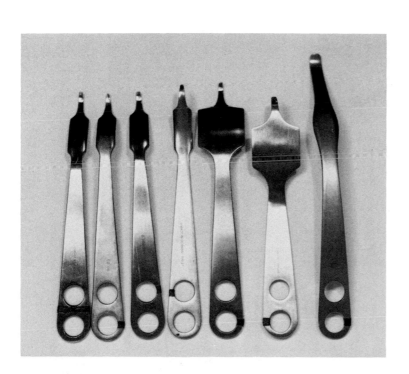

Figure 13–29. Hohmann retractors.

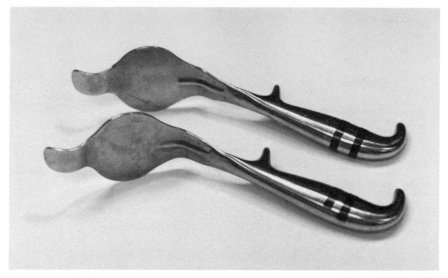

Figure 13–30. Bennett bone elevator retractors.

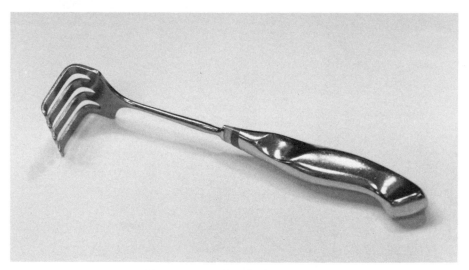

Figure 13–31. Israel rake retractor.

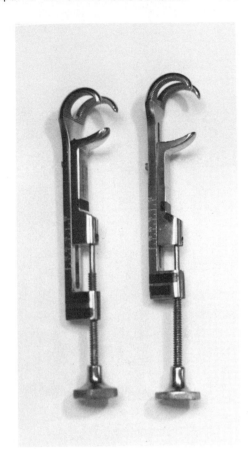

Figure 13–32. Lowman bone holding clamps.

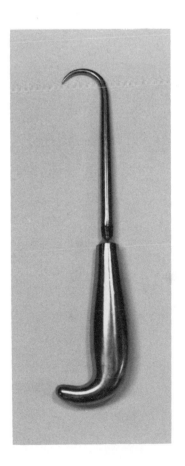

Figure 13–33. Bone hook.

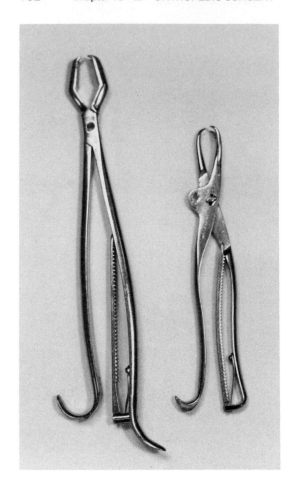

Figure 13–34. *Left.* Lane bone holding forcep. *Right.* Bishop bone clamp.

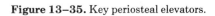

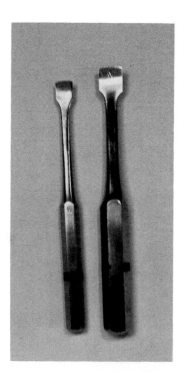

Figure 13–35. Key periosteal elevators.

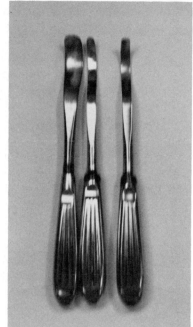

Figure 13–36. Crego periosteal elevators.

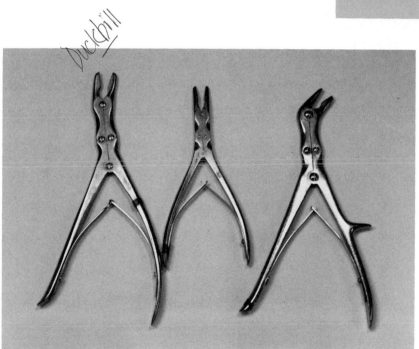

Figure 13–37. *Left to right.* Leksell bone rongeur, Jansen-Zaufel bone rongeur, and Echlin bone rongeur.

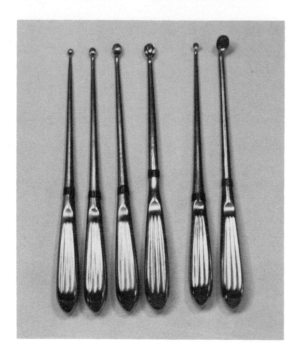

Figure 13–38. Brun bone curettes: straight and angled.

Figure 13–39. Ferris-Smith tissue forceps.

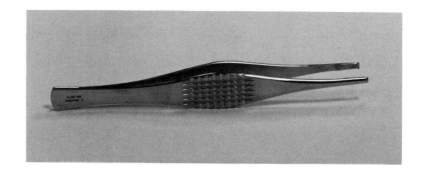

Figure 13–40. Bone chisel.

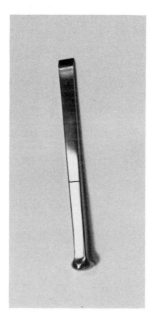

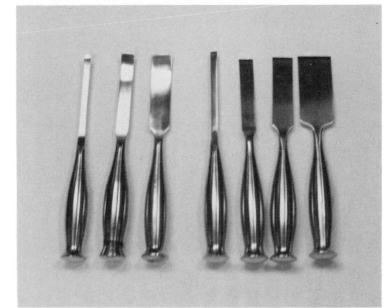

Figure 13–41. Smith-Peterson osteotomes: curved and straight.

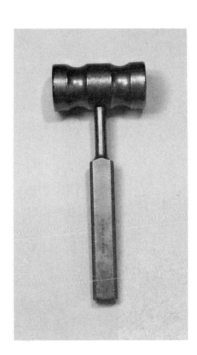

Figure 13–42. Zimmer bone mallet.

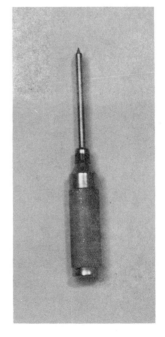

Figure 13–43. Zuelzer awl.

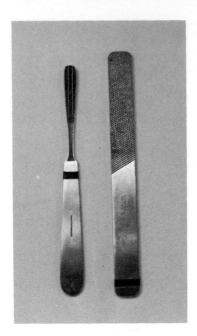

Figure 13–44. *Left.* Maltz nasal rasp. *Right.* Universal file.

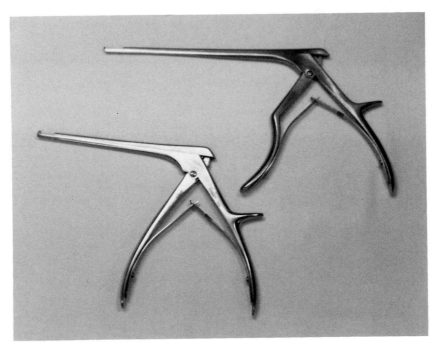

Figure 13–45. Kerrison cervical rongeurs.

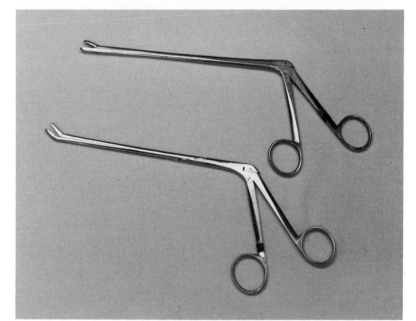

Figure 13–46. Cushing pituitary rongeurs: straight and curved.

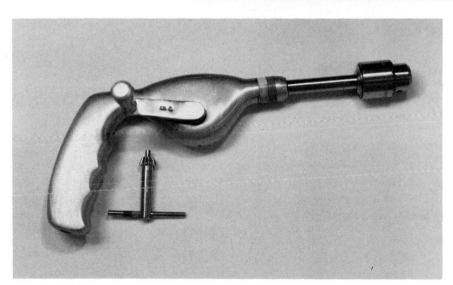

Figure 13–47. Hand drill with Jacobs chuck key.

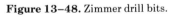

Figure 13–48. Zimmer drill bits.

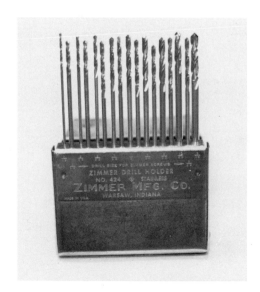

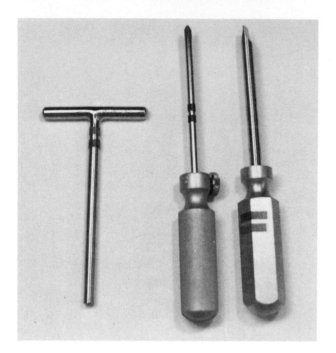

Figure 13–49. *Left to right.* T-wrench, Phillips screwdriver, and straight screwdriver.

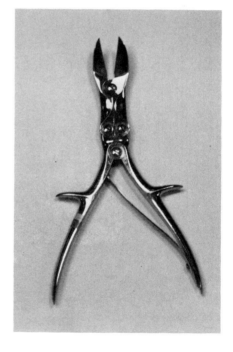

Figure 13–50. Stille-Horsley bone cutting forceps.

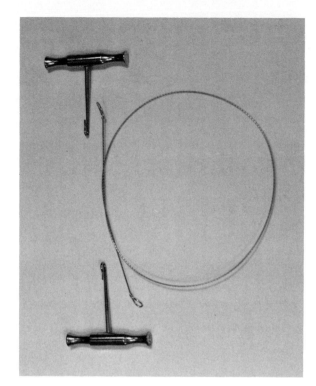

Figure 13–51. Solid Gigli saw handles with Gigli saw blade.

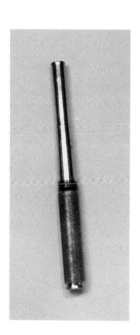

Figure 13–52. Kiene bone tamp

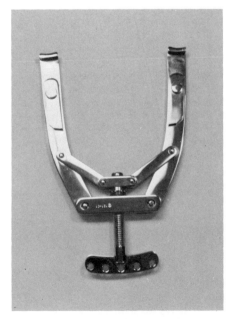

Figure 13–53. Traction bow.

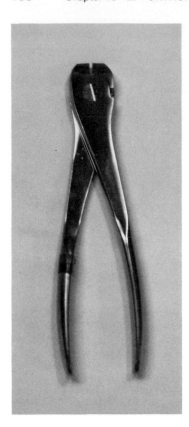

Figure 13–54. Wire cutter.

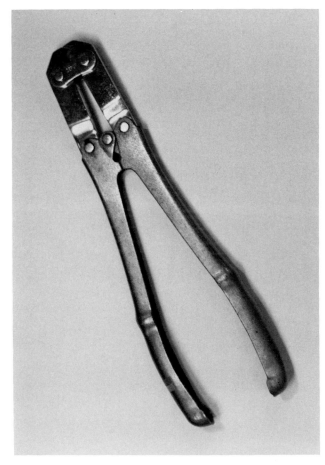

Figure 13–55. Multiaction pin cutter.

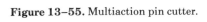

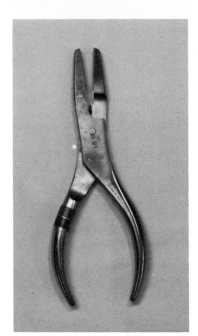

Figure 13–56. Needle-nosed pliers.

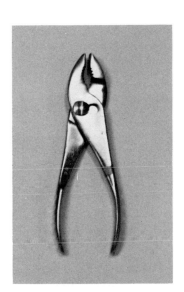

Figure 13–57. Standard pliers.

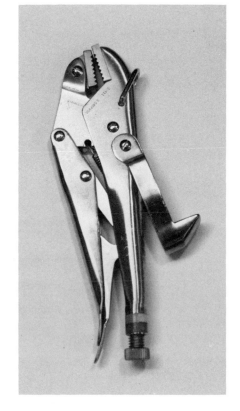

Figure 13–58. Vise-grip pliers.

Thoracic Surgery

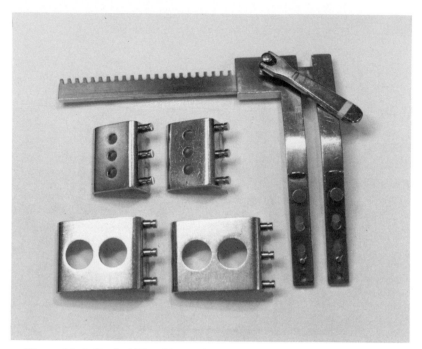

Figure 14–1. Burford-Finochietto rib spreader with interchangeable blades.

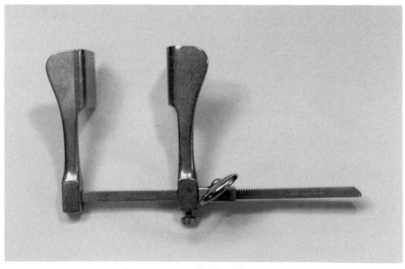

Figure 14–2. Tuffier rib spreader.

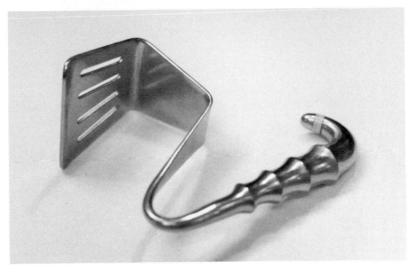

Figure 14–3. Davidson scapular retractor.

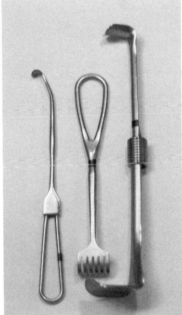

Figure 14–4. *Left to right.* Cushing vein retractor, 6-prong sharp Volkmann retractor, and double-ended Richardson retractor.

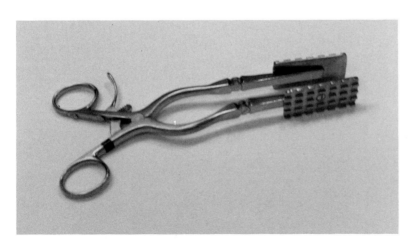

Figure 14–5. Ochsner vascular retractor.

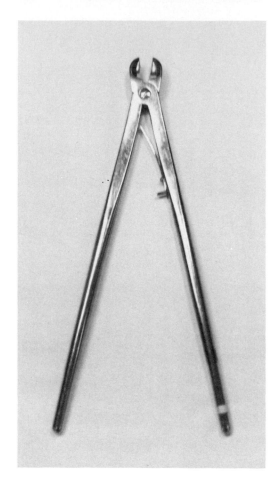

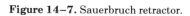
Figure 14–6. Bethune rib shears.

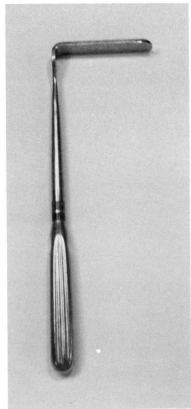

Figure 14–7. Sauerbruch retractor.

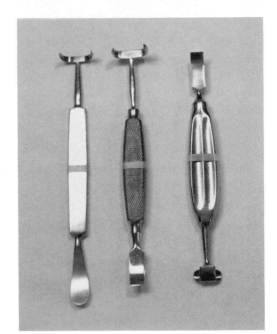

Figure 14–8. *Left to right.* Matson rib stripper and elevator, Matson-Alexander rib stripper and elevator, and Alexander double-ended costal periosteotome.

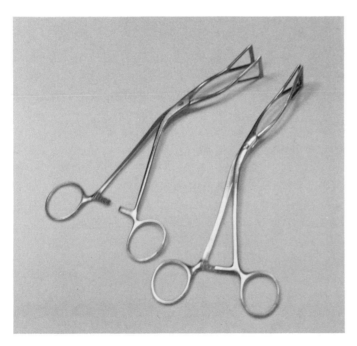

Figure 14–9. Lovelace lung forceps.

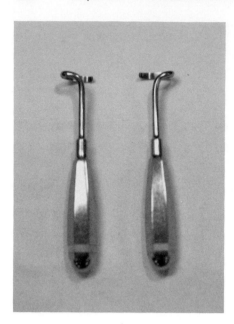

Figure 14–10. Doyen costal elevators: left and right blades.

Figure 14–11. Bailey rib contractor.

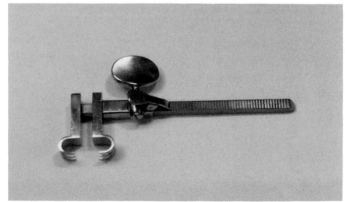

CHAPTER

15

Cardiovascular Surgery

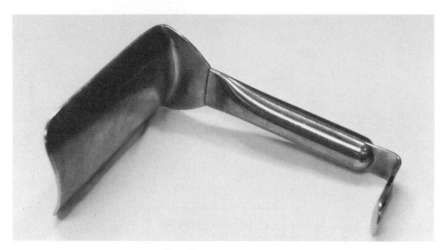

Figure 15–1. Weinberg vagotomy retractor (Joe's hoe).

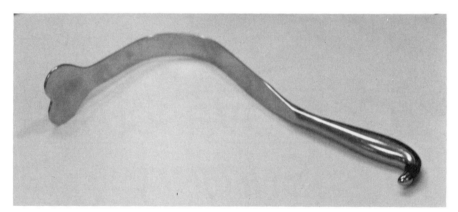

Figure 15–2. Harrington retractor.

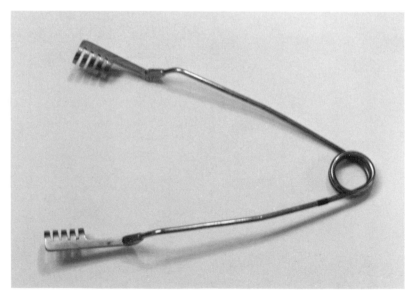

Figure 15–3. King goiter retractor.

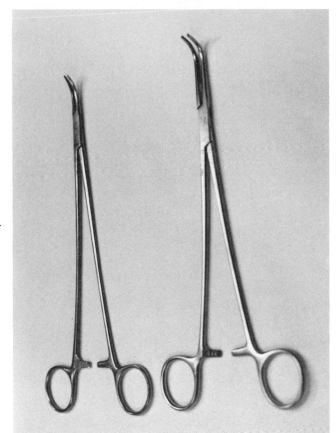

Figure 15–4. *Left.* Woodward thoracic artery forceps. *Right.* University of Michigan Mixter thoracic forceps.

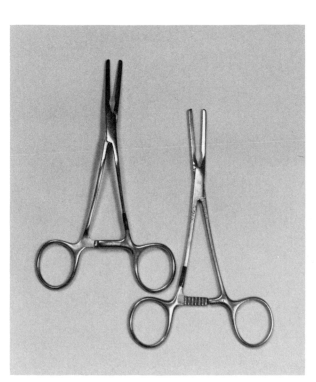

Figure 15–5. Cooley patent ductus clamps (straight jaw).

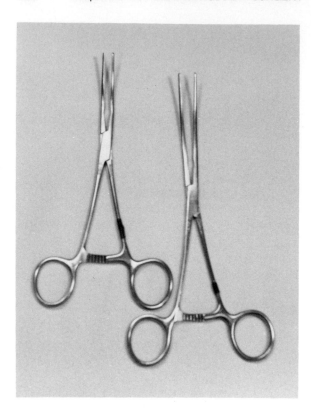

Figure 15–6. DeBakey-Bainbridge vascular clamps.

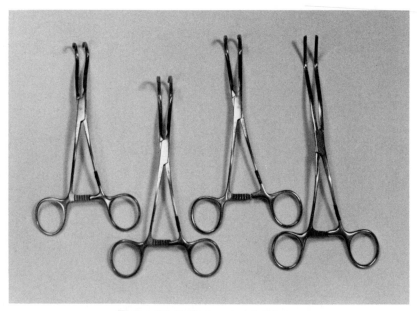

Figure 15–7. Cooley vascular clamps.

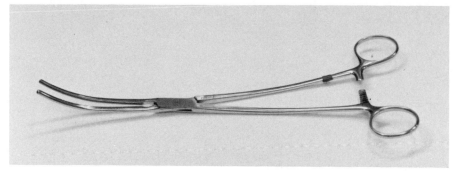

Figure 15–8. DeBakey aortic aneurysm clamp.

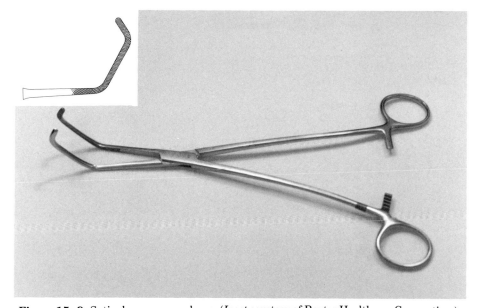

Figure 15–9. Satinsky vena cava clamp. (*Inset* courtesy of Baxter Healthcare Corporation.)

Figure 15–10. Cooley multipurpose clamp.

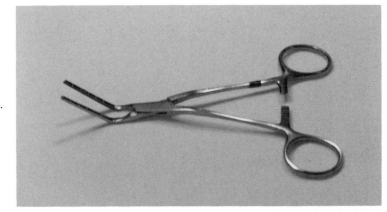

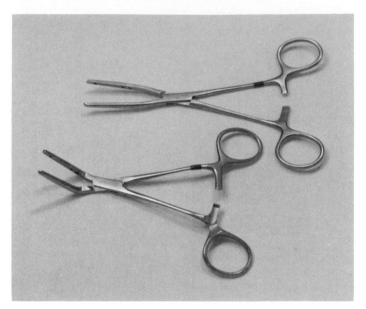

Figure 15–11. Fogarty clamps: angled and straight without inserts.

Figure 15–12. Javid artery bypass clamps.

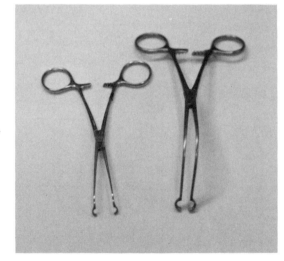

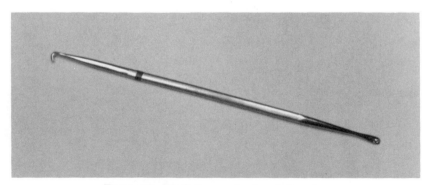

Figure 15–13. Crile nerve hook and dissector.

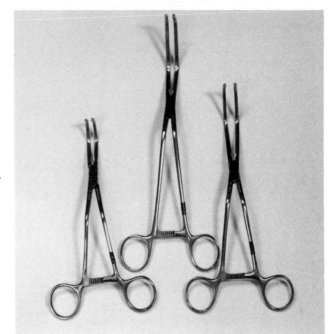

Figure 15–14. Bailey aortic clamps, various sizes.

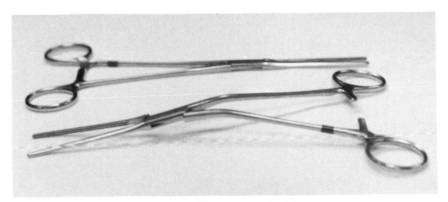

Figure 15–15. Glover coarctation clamps.

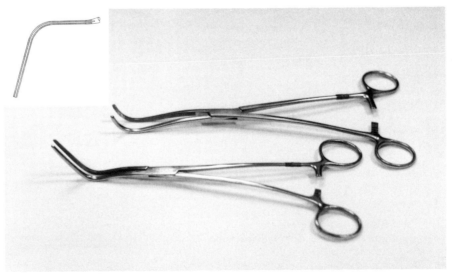

Figure 15–16. Harken auricle clamps Nos. 1 *(top)* and 4 *(bottom)*. (*Inset* courtesy of Baxter Health-care Corporation.)

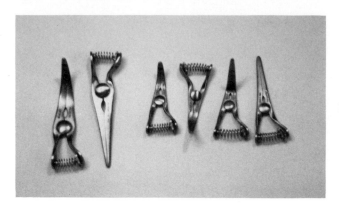

Figure 15–17. Glover bulldog clamps: straight and curved.

Figure 15–18. DeBakey bulldog clamps: straight and curved.

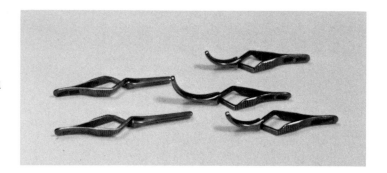

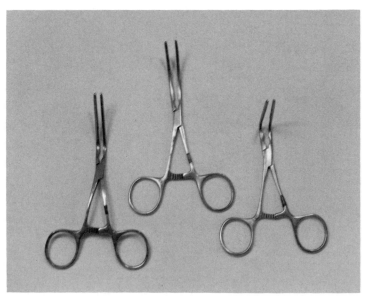

Figure 15–19. DeBakey bulldog clamps with ring handles.

Figure 15–20. Gregory bulldog clamp.

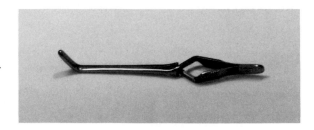

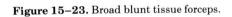

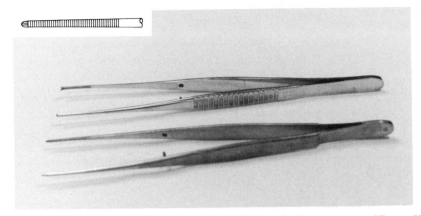

Figure 15–21. Potts-Smith tissue forceps with and without teeth. (*Inset* courtesy of Baxter Health-care Corporation.)

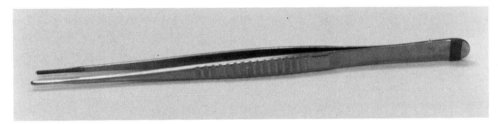

Figure 15–22. DeBakey tissue forceps.

Figure 15–23. Broad blunt tissue forceps.

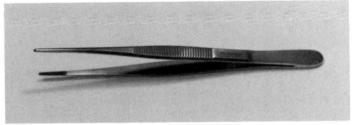

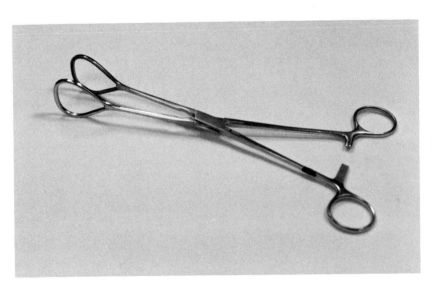

Figure 15–24. Stone trauma clamp.

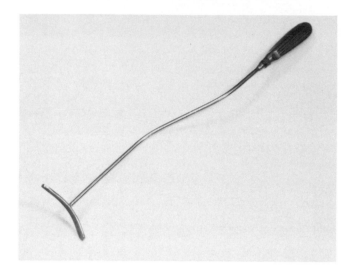

Figure 15–25. Conn aortic compressor.

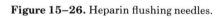

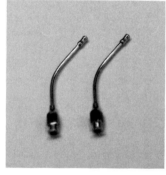

Figure 15–26. Heparin flushing needles.

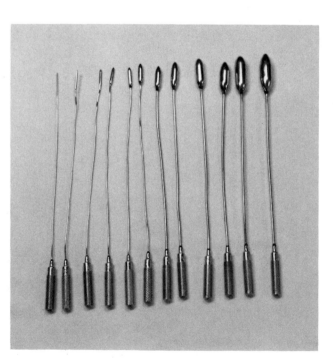

Figure 15–27. Garrett vascular dilators.

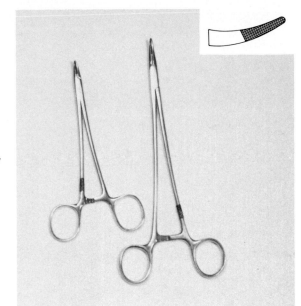

Figure 15–28. Julian needle holders. (*Inset* courtesy of Baxter Healthcare Corporation.)

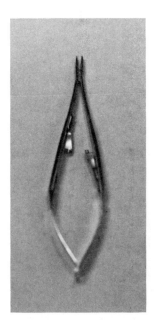

Figure 15–29. Castroviejo locking needle holder.

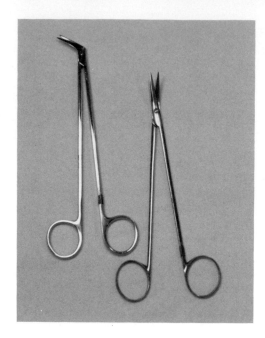

Figure 15–30. *Left.* Potts-Smith scissors. *Right.* DeMartel vascular scissors.

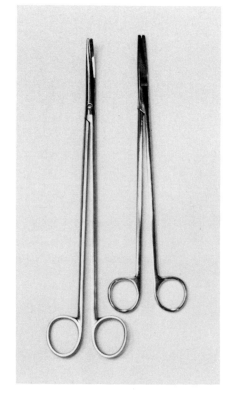

Figure 15–31. *Left.* Long Metzenbaum scissors. *Right.* Mayo-Harrington dissecting scissors.

Neurologic Surgery

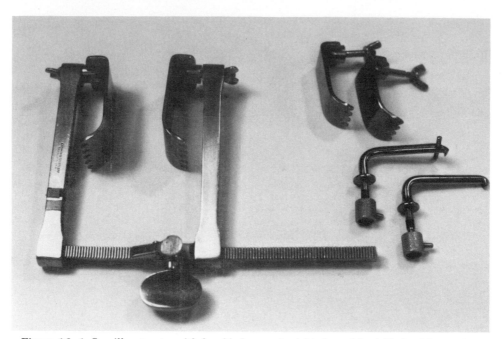

Figure 16–1. Scoville retractor with four blades, one hook blade, and hook blade with cross bar.

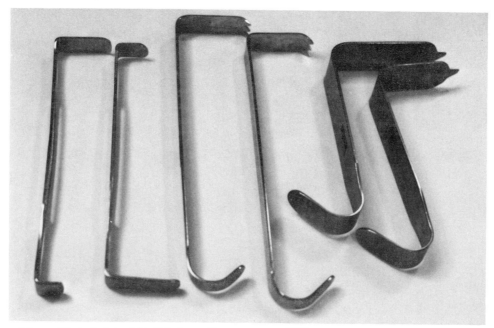

Figure 16–2. *Left to right.* U.S. Army-Navy retractors, Hibbs retractors, and Taylor retractors.

212

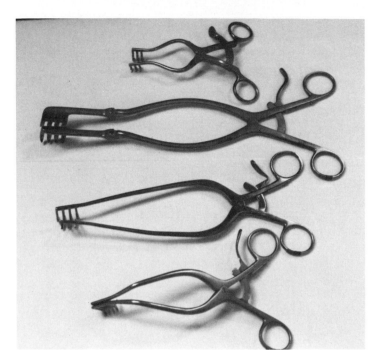

Figure 16–3. *Top to bottom.* Weitlaner retractor, Beckman retractor, Adson cerebellum retractor, and angled Adson cerebellum retractor.

Articulated —

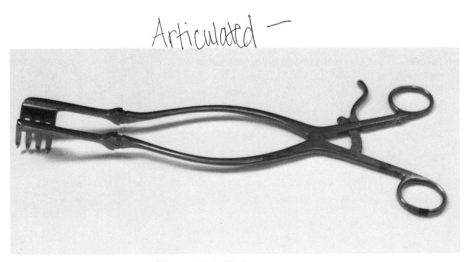

Figure 16–4. Beckman retractor.

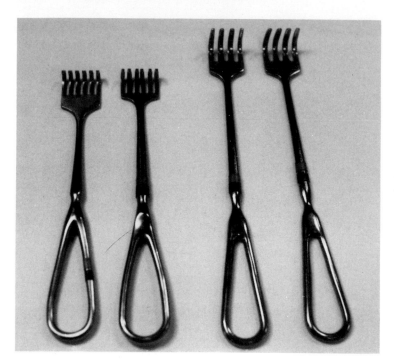

Figure 16–5. Volkmann retractors: two six-prong and two blunt four-prong.

Figure 16–6. *Left to right.* Love-Adson periosteal elevator, Lewin dissector, and Cushing elevator.

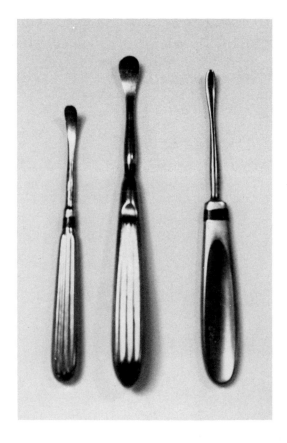

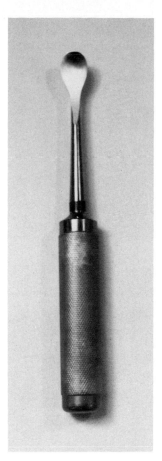

Figure 16–7. Cobb periosteal elevator.

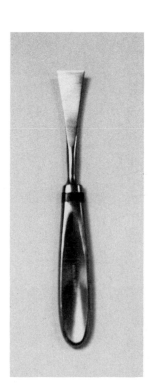

Figure 16–8. Langenbeck periosteal elevator.

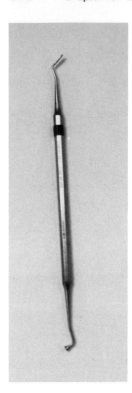

Figure 16–9. Woodson dural separator and packer.

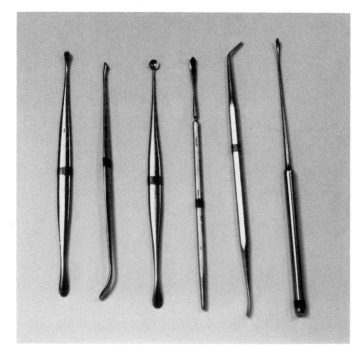

Figure 16–10. *Left to right.* Penfield dissectors Nos. 3, 2, 1; Davis nerve separator spatula; Crile knife and dissector; and Penfield dissector No. 4.

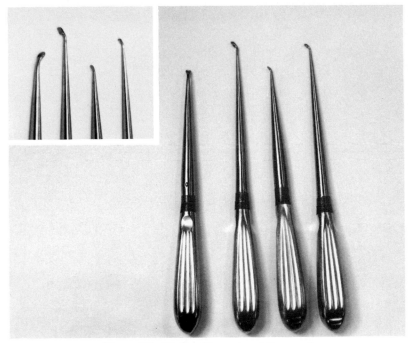

Figure 16–11. Scoville ruptured disc curettes.

Figure 16–12. *Left.* Bayonet tissue forceps. *Right.* Two tissue forceps with and without teeth.

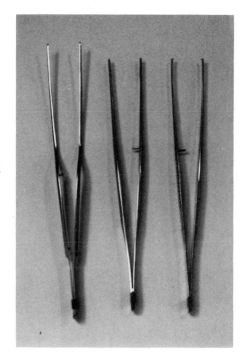

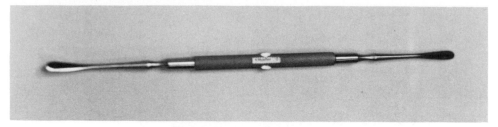

Figure 16–13. Freer elevator.

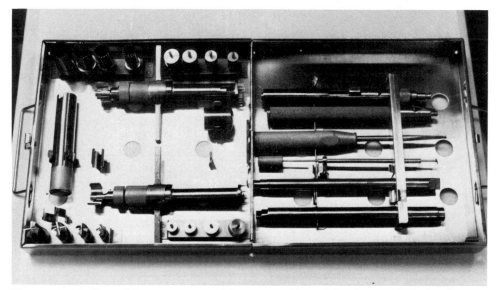

Figure 16–14. Cloward instrument case with contents: Cloward dowel cutter shaft, dowel ejector, osteophyte elevator, depth gauge, guard guide, dowel ejector pins, dowel cutter pins, cervical drill guards, drill guard cap, drill shaft, cervical drills, crossbar handle, dowel cutter shaft guard, and spanner wrench.

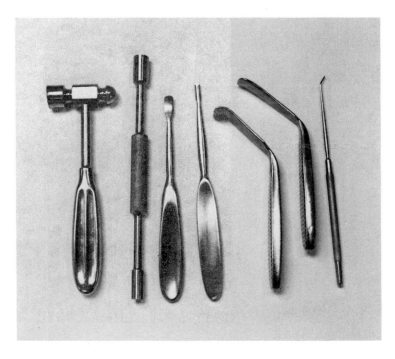

Figure 16–15. *Left to right.* Cloward hammer, Cloward bone graft impactor, double-ended; Cloward sharp periosteal elevator, Langenbeck periosteal elevator, Cloward blade retractors, and Cloward cautery hook.

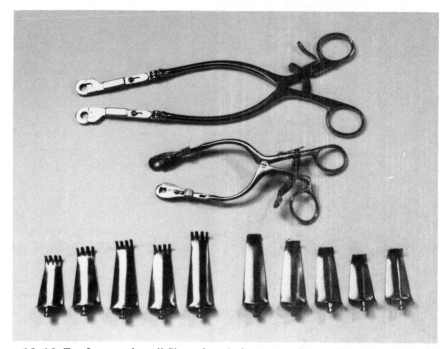

Figure 16–16. *Top.* Large and small Cloward cervical retractors. *Bottom.* Five Cloward sharp blades and five Cloward blunt blades.

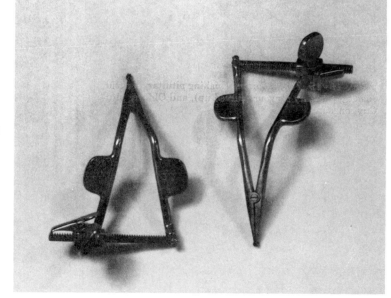

Figure 16–17. Cloward vertebra spreaders with ratchets.

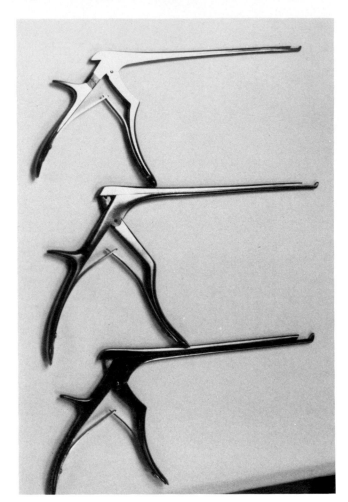

Figure 16–18. Kerrison cervical rongeurs.

Figure 16–19. *Top to bottom.* Cushing pituitary rongeur, Cushing pituitary rongeur (curved up), and Oldberg pituitary rongeur.

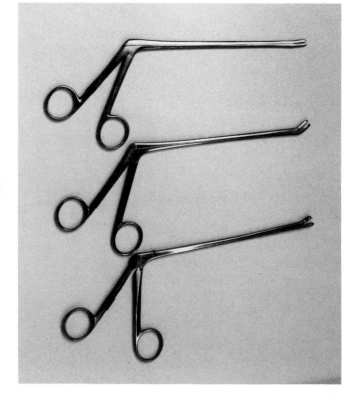

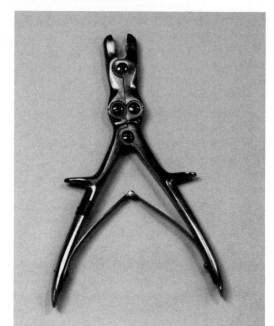

Figure 16–20. Stille-Luer rongeur.

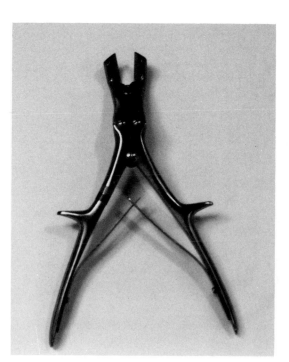

Figure 16–21. Horsley bone cutting forceps.

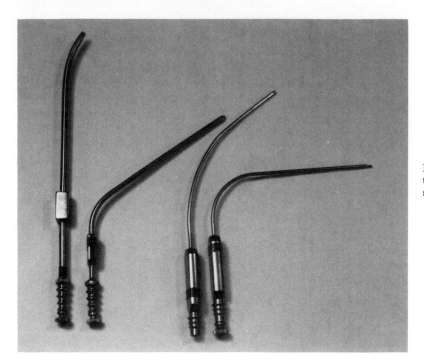

Figure 16–22. *Left to right.* Adson suction tube, Frazier suction tube, and two neurologic suction tips.

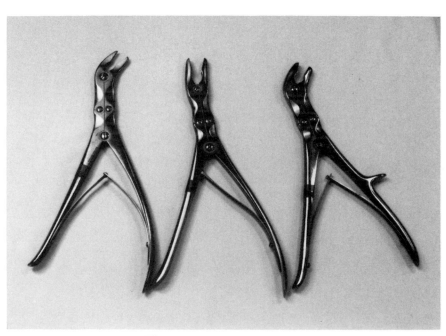

Figure 16–23. Leksell rongeurs.

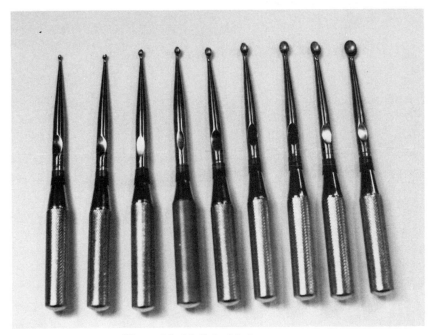

Figure 16–24. Spinal fusion curettes.

Figure 16–25. Scoville nerve retractor.

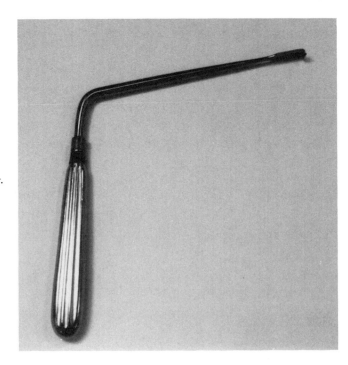

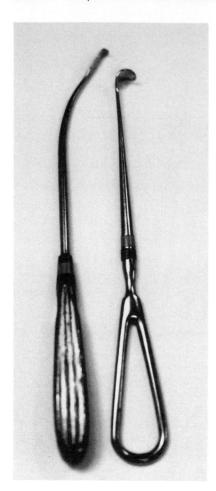

Figure 16–26. *Left.* Scoville nerve root retractor. *Right.* Cushing vein and nerve retractor.

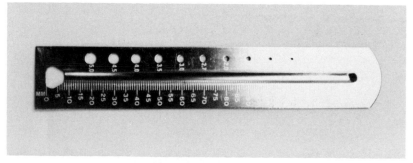

Figure 16–27. Zimmer ruler.

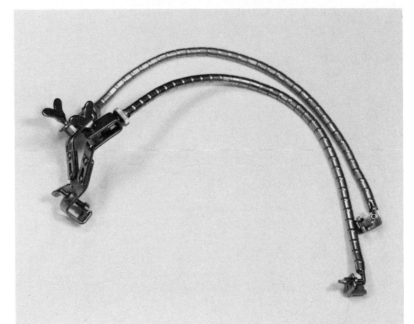

Figure 16–28. Leyla self-retaining brain retractor with flexible arms.

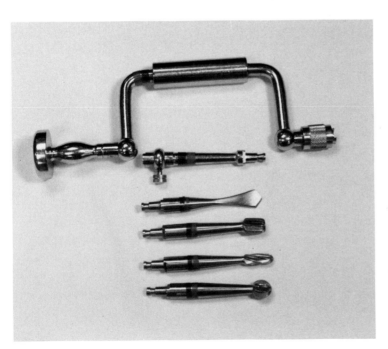

Figure 16–29. Hudson brace drill and accessories *(top to bottom):* Hudson cerebellar extension, Cushing perforator drill, and three Hudson burs.

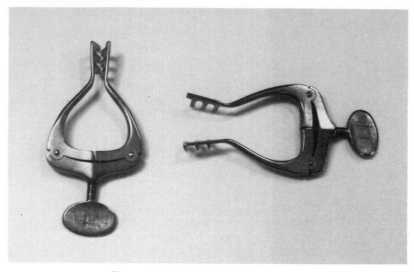

Figure 16–30. Jansen scalp retractors.

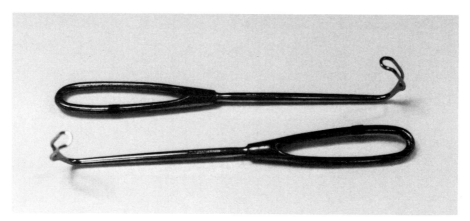

Figure 16–31. Cushing decompression retractors.

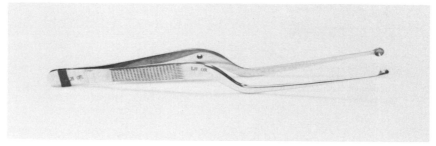

Figure 16–32. Adson hypophyseal forceps.

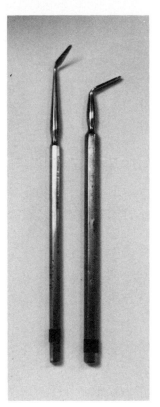

Figure 16–33. *Left.* Frazier dura elevator. *Right.* Frazier dura separator.

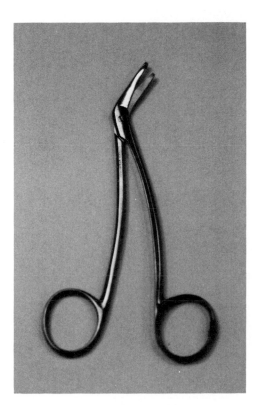

Figure 16–34. Taylor dural scissors.

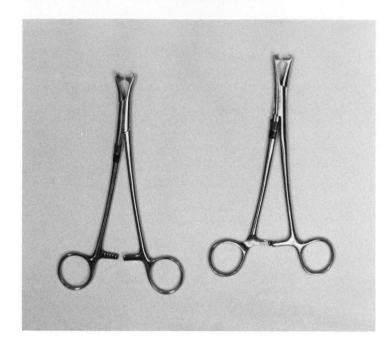

Figure 16–35. LeRoy clip appliers (adult and child).

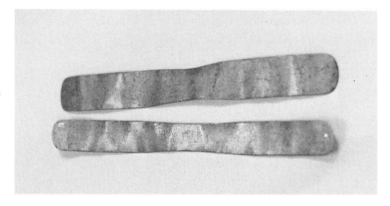

Figure 16–36. Mayfield brain spatulas (malleable).

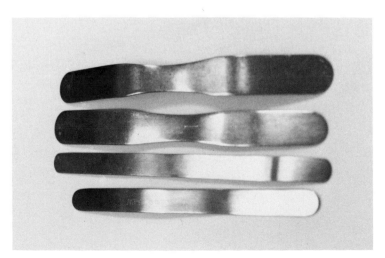

Figure 16–37. Davis brain retractors.

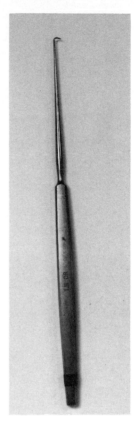

Figure 16–38. Adson dural hook.

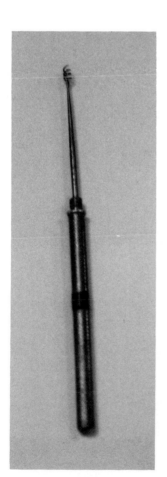

Figure 16–39. Corkscrew dural hook.

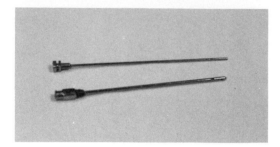

Figure 16–40. Cone ventricular needle with stylet.

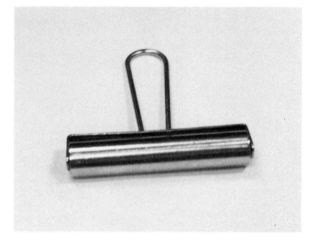

Figure 16–41. Spence cranioplastic roller.

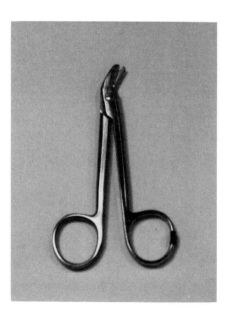

Figure 16–42. Wire scissors.

CHAPTER
17

Laser Surgery

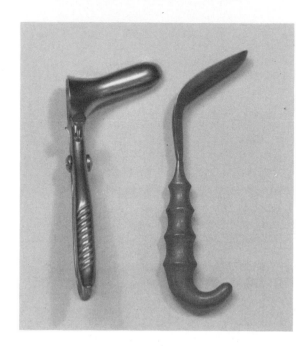

Figure 17–1. *Left.* Pratt rectal retractor. *Right.* Sawyer rectal retractor.

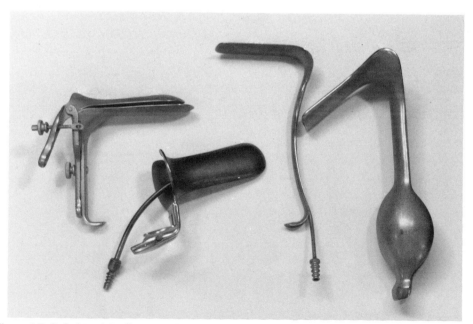

Figure 17–2. *Left to right.* Graves vaginal speculum, Collins vaginal speculum with suction, Jackson retractor with suction, and Auvard weighted speculum.

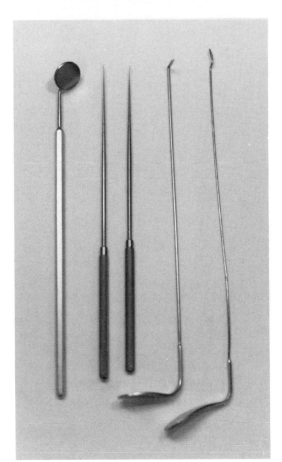

Figure 17–3. *Left to right.* Laser mirror with handle, two laser hooks, laser vaginal measuring rod, and lateral measuring rod (ruler).

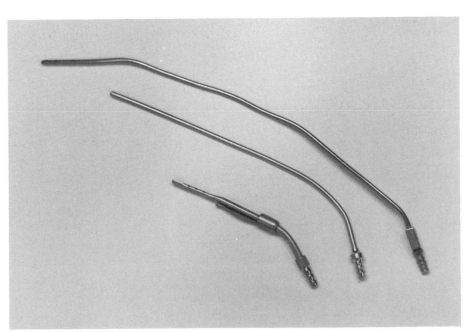

Figure 17–4. *Top to bottom.* Laser suction with hole, laser suction without hole, and short laser suction adapter.

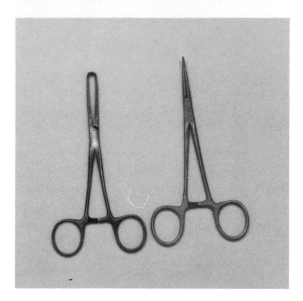

Figure 17–5. Laser Allis and Crile forceps.

Figure 17–6. Laser bayonet tissue forceps.

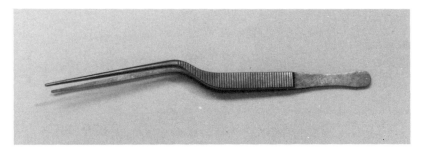

Index